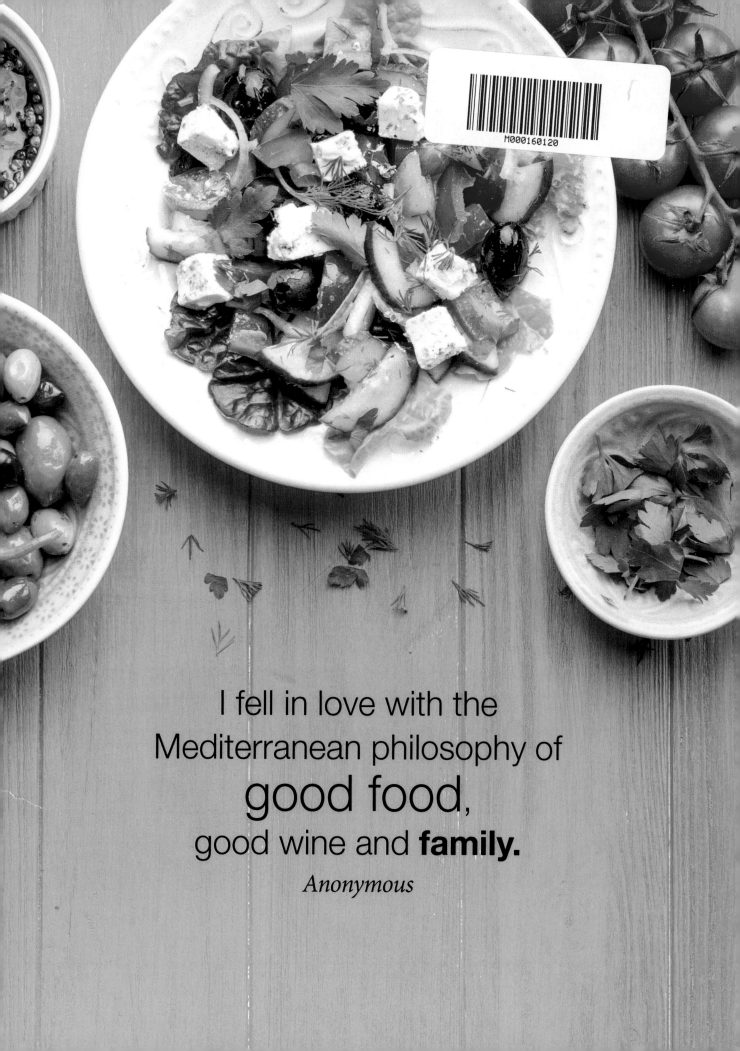

I fell in love with the
Mediterranean philosophy of
good food,
good wine and **family.**
Anonymous

INTRODUCTION

Summer is a wonderful time of year, full of sunshine and socializing! However, all those picnics, barbeques and parties can make it very difficult to stick to the keto diet. Surrounded with sandwiches, rolls, cakes and other high-carb treats, you may find your only keto options are a slab of overcooked meat and a scattering of salad…

This book is here to help and it is full of delicious, light and seasonal recipes with a Mediterranean twist. The Mediterranean diet is widely recognized as a very healthy diet with its emphasis on fresh produce and lots of olive oil, nuts and seafood. It also encourages the use of herbs and spices as opposed to salt to flavor food. The recipes in this book are low-carb dishes with flavors inspired by the cuisines of those in Greece, Italy, Spain and southern France.

With the warmer climate of summer and the inclination for more outdoor living, the keto diet can, at times, feel a bit heavy and too filling. Dealing with the heat and a more active lifestyle often lead to cravings for food that is light and fresh – and that is where the Mediterranean twist comes in. A traditional Mediterranean diet puts a great emphasis on fresh vegetables and seafood (although there are a great range of meat dishes included in this book too), which can fit really well into your already established keto diet as long as you stick with non-starchy vegetables. Adding more healthy fats-such as olive oil, avocados, and nuts, to your diet is something that also works well when following a ketogenic way of eating.

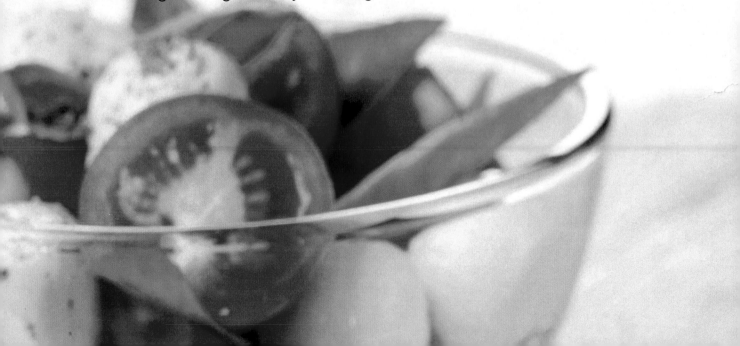

Here are some quick tips to eating keto in the summer, inspired by the Mediterranean way of life:

• Eat more (non-starchy) vegetables

• Eat more healthy fats

• Eat more fish and seafood

• Use herbs and spices to flavor food

• Put more emphasis on eating fresh produce

• Stick to seasonal vegetables as much as possible

• Take a "fresher" and "cleaner" approach to the keto diet

Many of the recipes included in this book are very portable so consider taking some of these delicious dishes along to the next picnic, barbeque or party you are invited to – they are guaranteed to be a hit! If you are feeling really sociable (and a little bit brave), you could even host your own keto picnic or barbeque!

I hope that the light and fresh recipes included in this book help you to stay on the keto track while making the most of all the long, beautiful days of summer.

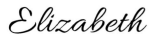

BONUS KETO SWEET EATS

I am delighted you have chosen my book to help you start or continue on your keto journey. Temptation by sweet treats can knock you off course so, to help you stay on the keto track, I am pleased to offer you three mini ebooks from my 'Keto Sweet Eats Series', completely free of charge! These three mini ebooks cover how to make everything from keto chocolate cake to keto ice cream to keto fat bombs so you don't have to feel like you are missing out, whatever the occasion.

Simply visit the link below to get your free copy of all three mini ebooks:

http://ketojane.com/summer

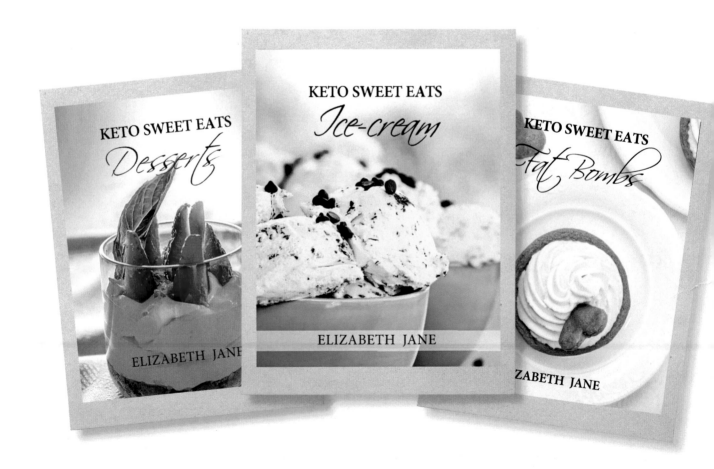

HOW THIS BOOK WORKS

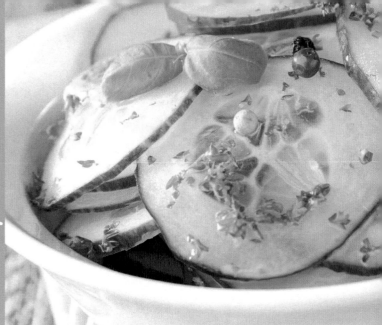

This cookbook contains helpful cooking tips to help you get the best results possible. There are also serving suggestions included to give you an idea about what each of these dishes pairs well with.

Each recipe starts with a guideline on the following:

Serves:
How many servings each recipe requires. This can be adjusted. For example, by doubling the quantity of all of the ingredients, you can make twice as many servings.

Difficulty Level:
1: An easy-to-make recipe that can be put together with just a handful of ingredients and in a short amount of time.

2: These recipes are a little more difficult and time consuming but are still easy enough even for beginners!

3: A more advanced recipe for the more adventurous cook! You will not see too many Level 3 recipes in this book. These recipes are great for when you have a little bit more time to spend in the kitchen and when you want to make something out of the ordinary.

Cost:
$: A low-budget everyday recipe.

$$: A middle-of-the-road, moderately priced recipe.

$$$: A more expensive recipe that is great for serving at a family gathering or party. These recipes tend to contain pricey ingredients, such as higher quality meat products.

Preparation Time:
Time required to prepare the recipe. This does not include the cooking time.

Cook Time:
Time required to cook the recipe. This does not include the preparation time.

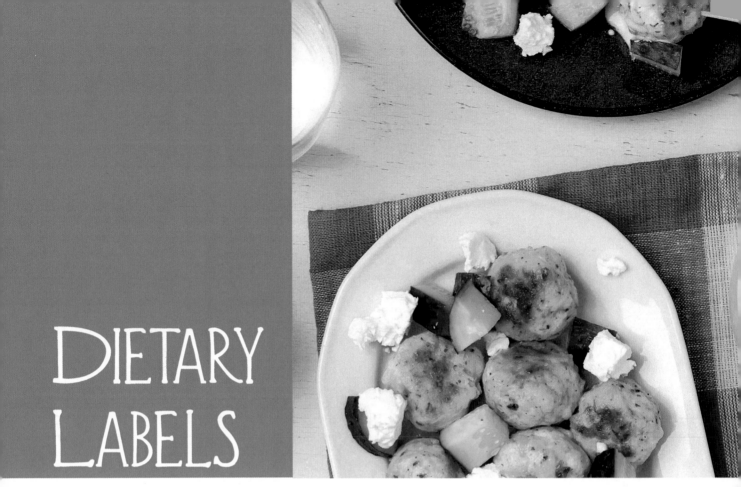

DIETARY LABELS

Within this book, you will notice that there are dietary labels. These will indicate whether a recipe is gluten-free, dairy-free or vegetarian. Please note that many recipes can be made dairy-free by removing the cheese in them or by substituting the milk or cream for coconut milk. Each recipe will also be labeled if it is gluten-free. Although the majority of the recipes are gluten-free, always be sure to check the food label on the ingredients you buy due to the variations in certain product ingredients.

GF: Gluten-free

DF: Dairy-free

V: Vegetarian (includes dairy products)

P: Paleo - (There are also Paleo substitutions for recipes that are not naturally Paleo friendly)

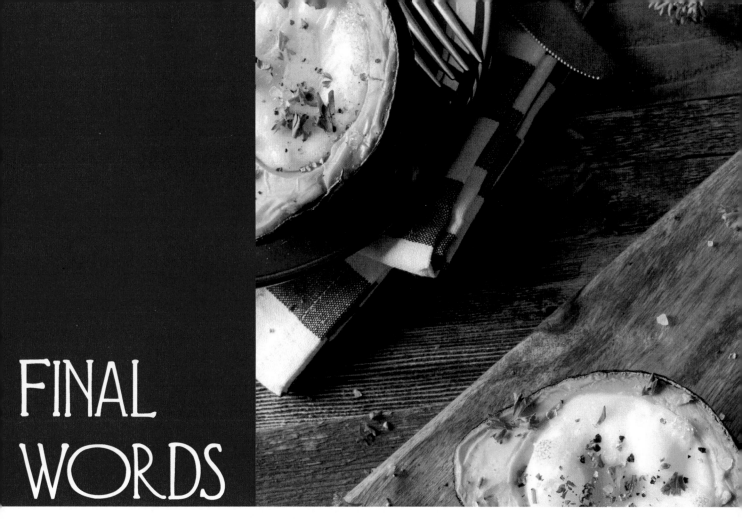

FINAL WORDS

Finally, I want to thank you for purchasing this book and I really hope it helps you keep to your health goals.

If you enjoyed this book or have any suggestions, then I'd appreciate it if you would leave a review or simply email me.

You can leave a review on Amazon at the link below,
or email me at: elizabeth@ketojane.com

To leave a review on Amazon, please visit:
http://ketojane.com/Summerreview

Elizabeth

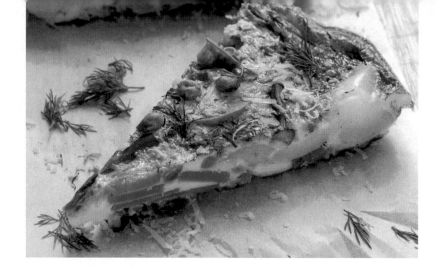

CONTENTS

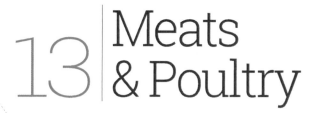

13 | Meats & Poultry

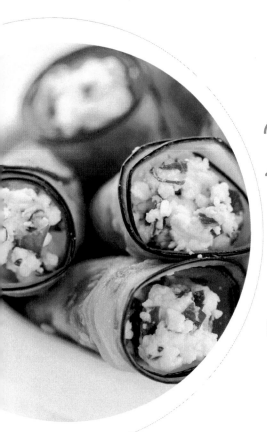

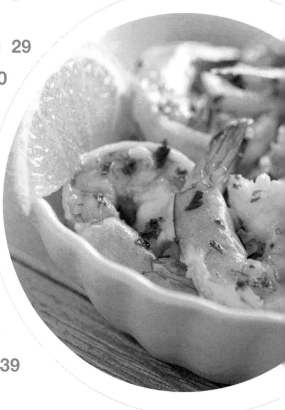

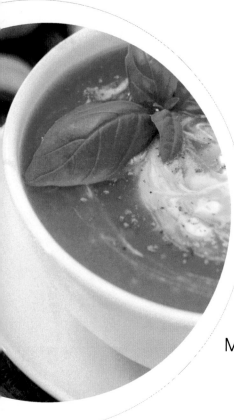

40 | Soups

49 | Salads

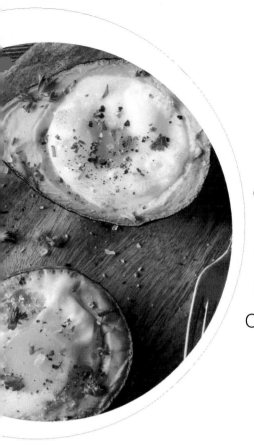

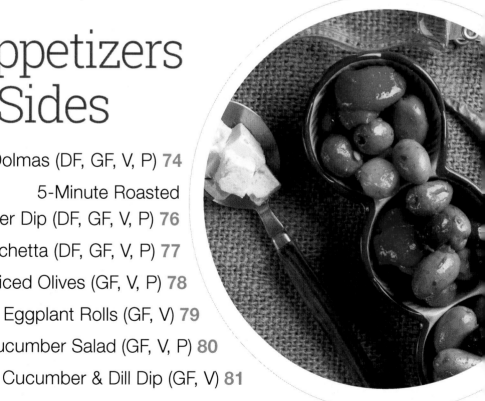

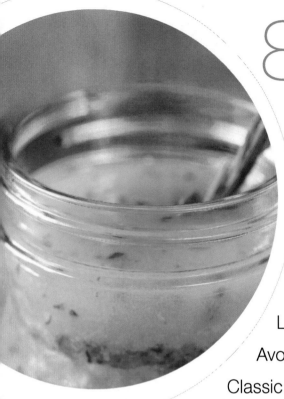

82 | Sauces & Dressing

93 | Desserts

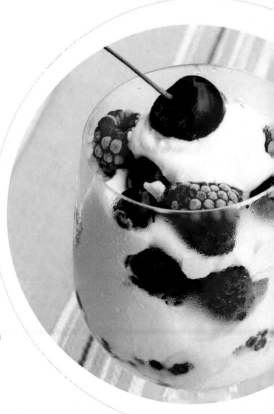

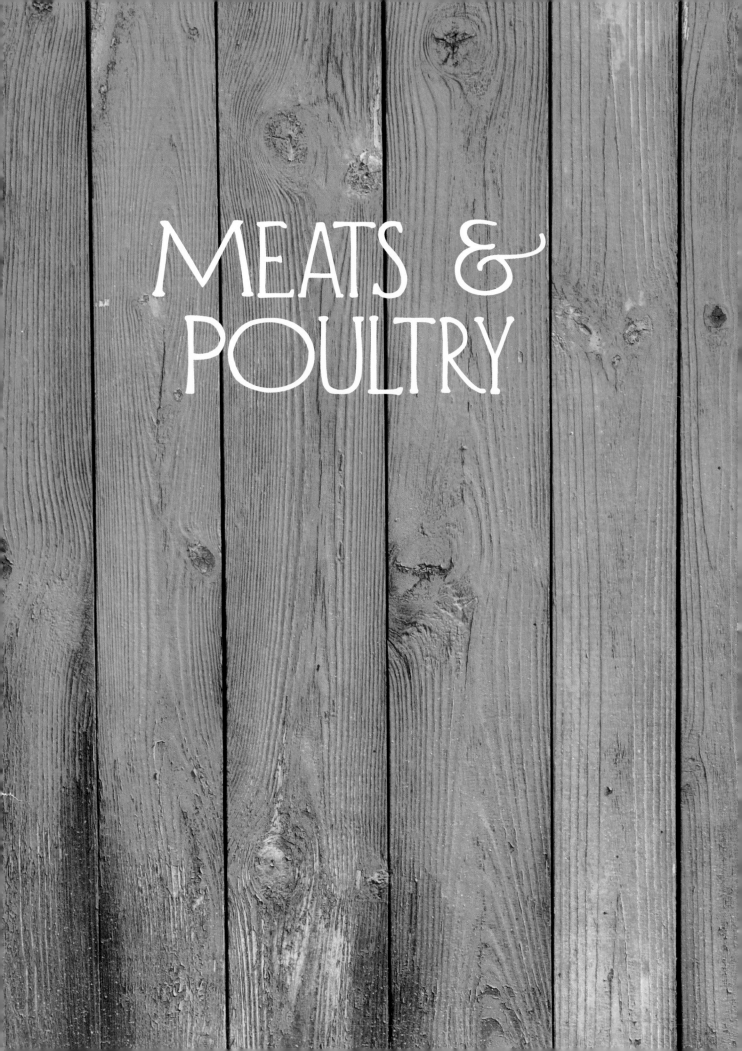

Meats & Poultry

TURKEY MEATBALLS WITH CUCUMBER YOGURT SAUCE GF

Serves: 6   Difficulty Level: 2   Cost: $$ Prep Time: 15 minutes
Cook Time: 15-20 minutes

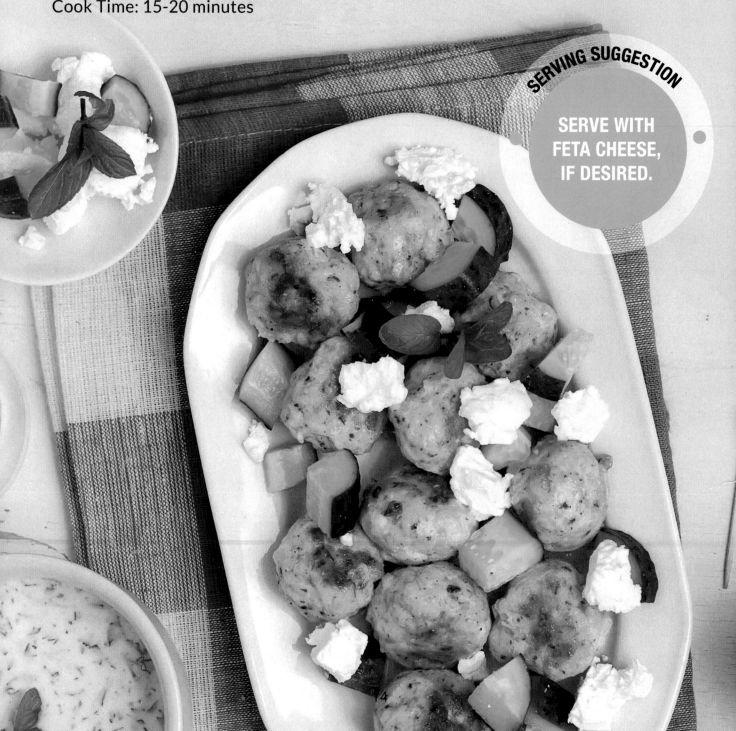

SERVING SUGGESTION

SERVE WITH FETA CHEESE, IF DESIRED.

Ingredients:

1 lb. ground turkey

1 egg

1 Tbsp. Italian seasoning

1 cup full-fat unsweetened Greek yogurt (use an unsweetened coconut based yogurt for a Paleo version)

1 cucumber, chopped

1 Tbsp. fresh dill

Salt & pepper to taste

Directions:

1. Start by preheating the oven to 375°F and lining a baking sheet with parchment paper.

2. Add the turkey, egg, Italian seasoning, salt and pepper to a mixing bowl. Stir to combine.

3. Form the turkey mixture into 12 medium sized meatballs and place them on the baking sheet. Bake for 15-20 minutes, turning halfway through. Increase by increments of 5 minutes if the turkey is not cooked through.

4. While the meatballs are cooking, make the sauce by stirring together the yogurt, cucumber and dill.

5. Drizzle the sauce over the meatballs and enjoy.

Nutrition Facts (Per Serving)

Calories: 209   Carbs: 4g   Fiber: 0g
Net Carbs: 4g   Protein: 25g   Fat: 12g

% calories from
Fat 48%   Carbs 7%   Protein 45%

GREEK GF STYLE BISON BURGER

Serves: 4   Difficulty Level: 2
Cost: $$ Prep Time: 10 minutes
Cook Time: 10-12 minutes

Ingredients:

1 lb. ground bison

½ cup crumbled feta cheese
(eliminate for a Paleo version)

1 Tbsp. freshly chopped dill

1 garlic clove, peeled and chopped

Salt & pepper to taste

Olive oil for cooking

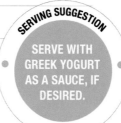

SERVING SUGGESTION

SERVE WITH GREEK YOGURT AS A SAUCE, IF DESIRED.

Directions:

1. Start by adding all of the ingredients to a large mixing bowl and stir to combine. Form into 4 large burgers.

2. Preheat a large skillet over medium heat with the olive oil and cook the burgers for 5-6 minutes on each side or until cooked through.

3. Serve with lettuce leaves for the bun.

Nutrition Facts (Per Serving)

Calories: 322   Carbs: 2g Fiber: 0g
Net Carbs: 2g   Protein: 30g   Fat: 21g

% calories from
Fat 60%   Carbs 3%   Protein 38%

GARLIC & PEPPER CHICKEN BREASTS GF DF P

Serves: 2
Difficulty Level: 1
Cost: $$
Prep Time: 10 minutes
Cook Time: 20 minutes

SERVING SUGGESTION

SERVE WITH LETTUCE AND TOMATOES, IF DESIRED.

Ingredients:

2 chicken breasts

1 Tbsp. olive oil

1 tsp. garlic powder

1 tsp. onion powder

1 tsp. ground peppercorns

Coconut oil for cooking

Directions:

1. Start by heating a grill pan over medium heat with the coconut oil.

2. While the pan is heating up, season the chicken with the olive oil, garlic powder, onion powder and peppercorns.

3. Cook for about 10 minutes on each side or until cooked through.

Nutrition Facts (Per Serving)
Calories: 159
Carbs: 2g
Fiber: 1g
Net Carbs: 1g
Protein: 20g
Fat: 7g

% calories from
Fat 42% Carbs 5% Protein 53%

MEDITERRANEAN CHICKEN & SALAD GF DF P

Serves: 1 Difficulty Level: 1 Cost: $$
Prep Time: 10 minutes   Cook Time: 20 minutes

SERVING SUGGESTION
SERVE WITH A BALSAMIC VINEGAR AND OLIVE OIL DRESSING.

Ingredients:

1 chicken breast

1 Tbsp. olive oil

1 tsp. garlic powder

¼ tsp. salt

2 cups mixed lettuce leaves

½ avocado, pitted and sliced

¼ cup capers

Coconut oil for cooking

Directions:

1. Start by heating a grill pan over medium heat with the coconut oil.

2. While the pan is heating up, season the chicken with the olive oil, garlic powder and salt.

3. Cook for about 10 minutes on each side or until cooked through.

4. Add the lettuce to a large mixing bowl with the avocado and capers. Top with the chicken breast and enjoy.

Nutrition Facts (Per Serving)
Calories: 407   Carbs: 15g   Fiber: 8g
Net Carbs: 7g   Protein: 30g   Fat: 29g

% calories from
Fat 59%   Carbs 14%   Protein 27%

LEMON ROASTED CHICKEN GF DF P

Serves: 6
Difficulty Level: 2
Cost: $$
Prep Time: 15 minutes
Cook Time: 40-42 minutes

SERVING SUGGESTION

SERVE WITH ROASTED ASPARAGUS OR STEAMED BROCCOLI.

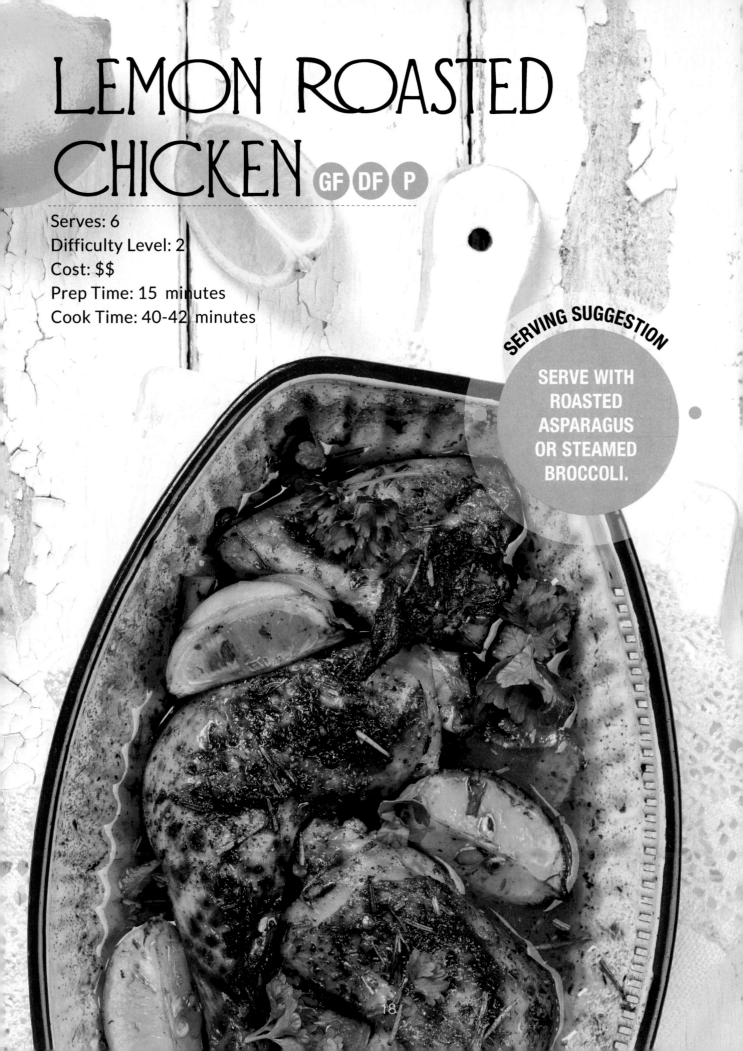

Ingredients:

6 chicken legs

2 garlic cloves, peeled and chopped

½ yellow onion, peeled and sliced

2 Tbsp. freshly squeezed lemon juice

4 lemon slices for garnish

1 tsp. dried oregano

1 tsp. fresh thyme (or more according to your taste)

¼ tsp. salt

¼ tsp. black pepper

Directions:

1. Start by preheating the oven to 425°F and greasing a baking dish with olive oil.

2. Next, add the chicken legs to the baking dish and season with the lemon juice, oregano, thyme, salt and pepper.

3. Add the garlic, onion and lemon slices to the baking dish.

4. Roast for 30 minutes or until the chicken legs begin to brown. Flip and then roast for an additional 10-12 minutes or until cooked through.

Nutrition Facts (Per Serving)

Calories: 167   Carbs: 7g   Fiber: 1g
Net Carbs: 6g   Protein: 10g   Fat: 11g

% calories from
Fat 59%   Carbs 17%   Protein 24%

MEDITERRA-NEAN FUSION STEAK (GF) (DF) (P)

Serves: 4 Difficulty Level: 2
Cost: $$ Prep Time: 20 minutes
Cook Time: 10-20 minutes

SERVING SUGGESTION
SERVE WITH FRESH GREENS OF YOUR CHOICE.

Ingredients:

2 lbs. flank steak

2 Tbsp. olive oil

2 Tbsp. fresh rosemary, chopped

1 Tbsp. capers

Salt & pepper to taste

Olive oil for cooking

Directions:

1. Start by marinating the steak with 2 tablespoons of olive oil, rosemary, salt and pepper. Allow this to marinate for 15 minutes.

2. Preheat a large skillet over medium heat with the olive oil reserved for cooking and cook the steak for 5-10 minutes on each side or until cooked to your liking.

3. Serve with capers.

Nutrition Facts (Per Serving)

Calories: 506 Carbs: 1g Fiber: 1g
Net Carbs: 0g Protein: 63g Fat: 26g

% calories from
Fat 48%   Carbs 1%   Protein 51%

ROSEMARY & PEPPER CHICKEN CUTLETS

Serves: 6
Difficulty Level: 2
Cost: $$
Prep Time: 15 minutes
Cook Time: 20 minutes

GF DF P

SERVING SUGGESTION

MAKE A CHICKEN
SANDWICH USING
LETTUCE LEAVES
AS THE "BREAD",
IF DESIRED.

Ingredients:

1 lb. ground chicken

½ cup almond flour

2 eggs

1 garlic clove, peeled and chopped

1 tsp. crushed peppercorns

2 Tbsp. coconut oil

1 tsp. fresh rosemary, chopped

1 tsp. garlic powder

1 tsp. onion powder

¼ tsp. salt

¼ tsp. black pepper

Nutrition Facts (Per Serving)
Calories: 222
Carbs: 2g
Fiber: 1g
Net Carbs: 1g
Protein: 24g
Fat: 13g

% calories from
Fat 53%
Carbs 4%
Protein 43%

Directions:

1. Start by adding the ground chicken to a large mixing bowl with the chopped garlic and mix to combine. Form into 12 small patties and set aside.

2. Next, add the almond flour, peppercorns, rosemary, garlic powder, onion powder, salt and pepper to a mixing bowl. Stir to combine.

3. Add the eggs to a large mixing bowl and whisk.

4. Next, dip each patty into the egg mixture, followed by the almond flour and seasoning mixture. Be sure to cover both sides of each patty with the almond flour mixture.

5. Allow the patties to sit for about 5 minutes.

6. Preheat a large skillet over medium heat with the coconut oil and cook each chicken patty for about 10 minutes on each side or until cooked through and browned.

7. Serve with mayonnaise, if desired.

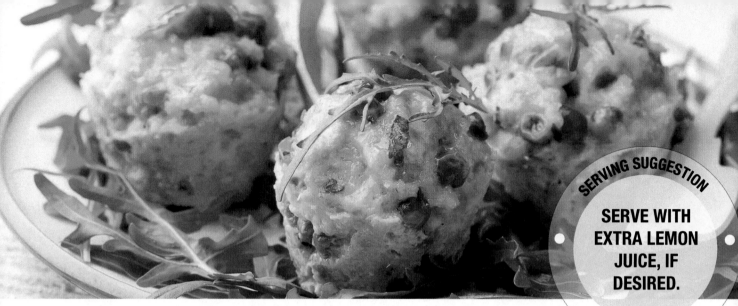

SERVING SUGGESTION

SERVE WITH EXTRA LEMON JUICE, IF DESIRED.

Serves: 6
Difficulty Level: 2
Cost: $$
Prep Time: 15 minutes
Cook Time: 15-20 minutes

Ingredients:

1 lb. ground turkey

1 egg

1 Tbsp. oregano

¼ cup green onion, chopped

2 Tbsp. freshly squeezed lemon juice

Salt & pepper to taste

Fresh arugula (for serving, optional)

Nutrition Facts
(Per Serving)

Calories: 163
Carbs: 1g
Fiber: 1g
Net Carbs: 0g
Protein: 22g
Fat: 9g

% calories from
Fat 47%   Carbs 2%
Protein 51%

LEMON & GREEN ONION TURKEY MEAT-BALLS

GF **DF** **P**

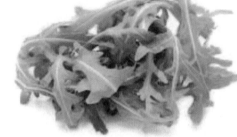

Directions:

1. Start by preheating the oven to 375°F and lining a baking sheet with parchment paper.

2. Add the turkey, egg, oregano, chopped green onion, lemon juice, salt and pepper to a mixing bowl. Stir to combine.

3. Form the turkey mixture into 12 medium sized meatballs and place them on the baking sheet. Bake for 15-20 minutes, turning halfway through. Increase by increments of 5 minutes if the turkey is not cooked through.

4. Once cooked, serve with fresh arugula, if desired.

VEGETARIAN RECIPES

SAUTÉED SUMMER VEGETABLES

Serves: 3
Difficulty Level: 1
Cost: $$
Prep Time: 10 minutes
Cook Time: 10 minutes

GF P DF V

SERVING SUGGESTION

SERVE WITH A SIDE SALAD, IF DESIRED.

Ingredients:

1 red bell pepper, cored and sliced

1 yellow bell pepper, cored and sliced

1 orange bell pepper, cored and sliced

1 cup button mushrooms

2 garlic cloves, peeled and chopped

1 red onion, peeled and quartered

3 Tbsp. olive oil

Salt & pepper to taste

Directions:

1. Start by heating a large skillet over medium heat with the olive oil. Add all of the chopped and sliced vegetables and sauté for about 10 minutes or until the vegetables are tender.

2. Season with salt and pepper and enjoy.

Nutrition Facts (Per Serving)

Calories: 181
Carbs: 14g
Fiber: 3g
Net Carbs: 11g
Protein: 3g
Fat: 14g

% calories from
Fat 65%
Carbs 29%
Protein 6%

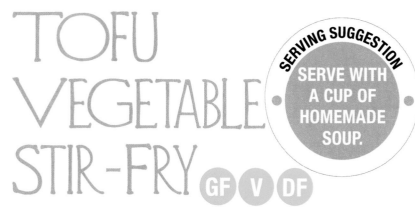

TOFU VEGETABLE STIR-FRY GF V DF

SERVING SUGGESTION SERVE WITH A CUP OF HOMEMADE SOUP.

Serves: 3   Difficulty Level: 1
Cost: $$ Prep Time: 10 minutes   Cook Time: 12 minutes

Ingredients:

1 cup tofu, drained, pressed and cut into cubes (use chicken for a Paleo version)

1 cup broccoli florets

½ cup eggplant, sliced

1 yellow bell pepper, cored and sliced

1 orange bell pepper, cored and sliced

¼ cup frozen peas

1 Tbsp. shallot, peeled and chopped

2 garlic cloves, peeled and chopped

3 Tbsp. olive oil

Salt & pepper to taste

Directions:

1. Start by heating a large skillet over medium heat with the olive oil. Add the cubed tofu and cook for about 7 minutes or until lightly brown.

2. Add in the remaining ingredients and sauté for another 5 minutes or until the vegetables are tender.

3. Season with salt and pepper and enjoy.

Nutrition Facts (Per Serving)

Calories: 276   Carbs: 11g   Fiber: 4g   Net Carbs: 7g
Protein: 15g Fat: 21g

% calories from   Fat 66%   Carbs 15%   Protein 15%

CHEESY BAKED EGGPLANT

Serves: 2
Difficulty Level: 1
Cost: $$
Prep Time: 15 minutes
Cook Time: 30 minutes

Ingredients:

1 eggplant, halved

½ cup shredded mozzarella cheese (eliminate for a Paleo version)

½ cup black olives, pitted and chopped

1 tomato, chopped

1 Tbsp. olive oil

1 tsp. dried oregano

Salt & pepper to taste

Directions:

1. Start by preheating the oven to 400°F and lining a baking sheet with parchment paper.

2. Add the eggplant halves onto the baking sheet and drizzle with olive oil.

3. Season with the salt, pepper and oregano, and top with the tomato, shredded cheese and chopped olives.

4. Bake for 30 minutes or until the cheese has melted and is lightly brown.

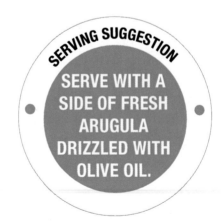

SERVING SUGGESTION

SERVE WITH A SIDE OF FRESH ARUGULA DRIZZLED WITH OLIVE OIL.

Nutrition Facts
(Per Serving)

Calories: 184
Carbs: 18g
Fiber: 10g
Net Carbs: 8g
Protein: 5g
Fat: 12g

% calories from
Fat 54%   Carbs 36%   Protein 10%

REFRESHING SUMMER NOODLES

Seafood Recipes

Serves: 2
Difficulty Level: 1
Cost: $$
Prep Time: 10 minutes
Cook Time: 5 minutes

Ingredients:

2 zucchinis, spiralized

8 cherry tomatoes, halved

1 garlic clove, peeled and chopped

1 Tbsp. crumbled feta cheese (eliminate for a Paleo version)

1 Tbsp. olive oil

Salt & pepper to taste

Nutrition Facts
(Per Serving)

Calories: 112
Carbs: 9g
Fiber: 3g
Net Carbs: 6g
Protein: 3g
Fat: 8g

% calories from
Fat 60%
Carbs 30%
Protein 10%

Directions:

1. Start by heating a large skillet over medium heat with the olive oil. Add the zucchini, garlic and tomatoes. Cook for about 5 minutes or until the zucchini is tender.

2. Serve with the crumbled feta cheese and season with salt and pepper.

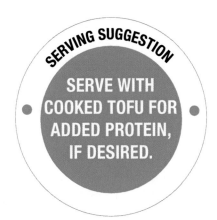

SERVING SUGGESTION

SERVE WITH COOKED TOFU FOR ADDED PROTEIN, IF DESIRED.

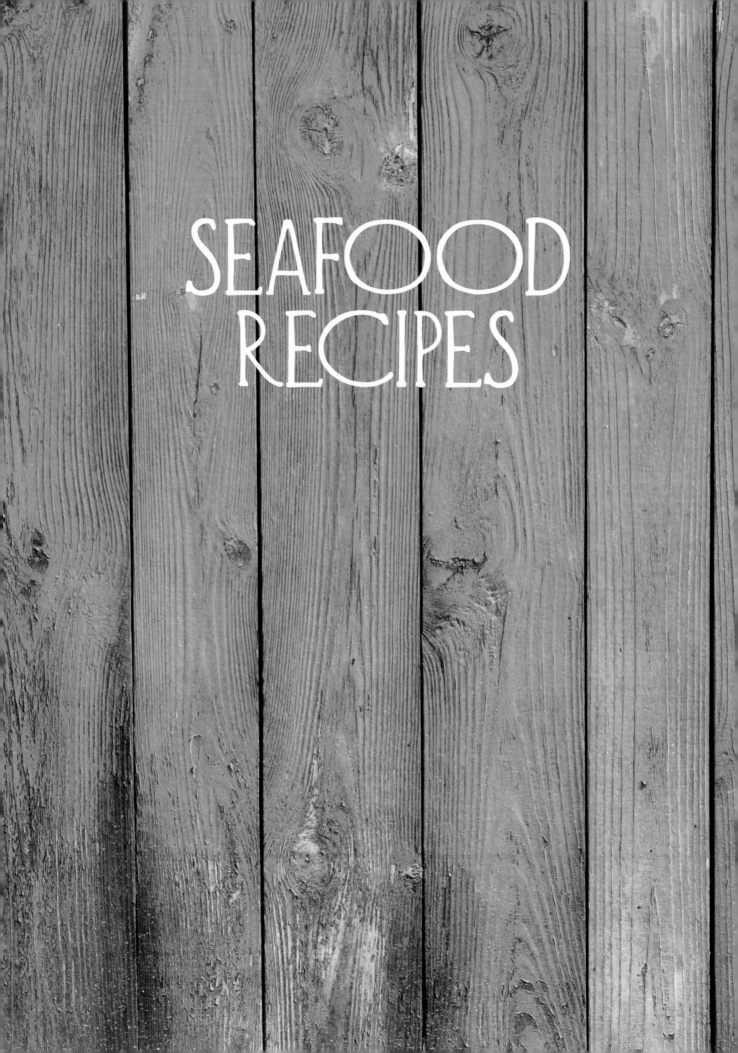

SEAFOOD RECIPES

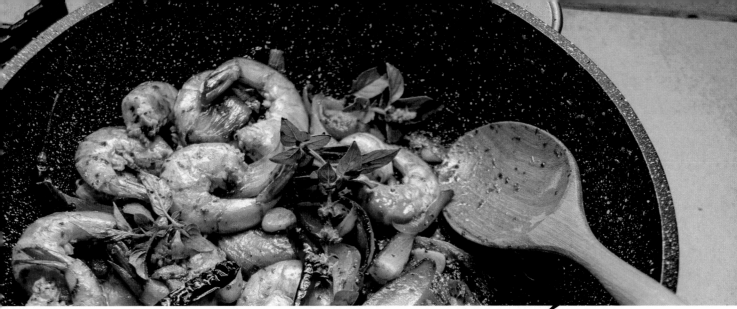

Serves: 3
Difficulty Level: 1
Cost: $$
Prep Time: 5 minutes
Cook Time: 6-9 minutes

HERB SAUTÉED SHRIMP (GF) (DF) (P)

Ingredients:

24 jumbo shrimp, peeled and deveined (tail left on)

2 Tbsp. olive oil

1 sprig fresh thyme

1 Tbsp. fresh mint leaves

½ yellow onion, peeled and thinly sliced

2 whole garlic cloves, peeled

½ tsp. salt

½ tsp. pepper

Directions:

1. Start by heating a large skillet over low-medium heat with the olive oil.

2. Add the shrimp and cook for about 4-5 minutes or until pink.

3. Add in the remaining ingredients and cook for another 2-3 minutes.

4. Transfer to a serving bowl and enjoy.

Nutrition Facts
(Per Serving)

Calories: 301
Carbs: 5g
Fiber: 1g
Net Carbs: 4g
Protein: 41g
Fat: 12g

% calories from

Fat 37%
Carbs 7%
Protein 56%

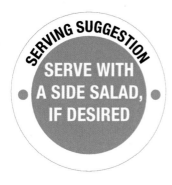

SERVING SUGGESTION
SERVE WITH A SIDE SALAD, IF DESIRED

SPICY MEDITERRANEAN SALMON BURGERS

GF

Serves: 4
Difficulty Level: 2
Cost: $$
Prep Time: 20 minutes
Cook Time: 6-8 minutes

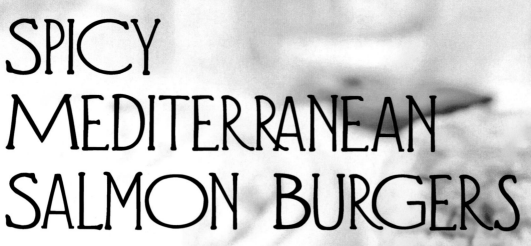

SERVING SUGGESTION

SERVE OVER
A BED OF FRESH
SPINACH,
IF DESIRED

Ingredients:

1 lb. salmon fillet (skin and bones removed)

1 Tbsp. mayonnaise
(use an avocado based or Paleo friendly mayonnaise for a Paleo version)

1 cup fresh spinach

1 garlic clove, peeled and chopped

1 jalapeño pepper, chopped

Salt & pepper to taste

1 avocado, pitted and cubed

2 Tbsp. unsweetened full-fat Greek yogurt (use an unsweetened coconut based yogurt for a Paleo version)

1 Tbsp. fresh dill

Olive oil for cooking

Directions:

1. Start by adding all of the ingredients, minus the avocado and Greek yogurt, to a food processor and process until smooth. Form into 4 burger patties.

2. Preheat a large skillet over medium heat with the olive oil and cook the burgers for 3-4 minutes each side or until cooked through.

3. While the burgers are cooking, make the avocado sauce by adding the avocado, dill and Greek yogurt to a food processor. Blend until smooth.

4. Top the burgers with the sauce and enjoy.

Nutrition Facts (Per Serving)
Calories: 278   Carbs: 7g   Fiber: 4g   Net Carbs: 3g   Protein: 24g   Fat: 18g
% calories from   Fat 57%   Carbs 10%   Protein 34%

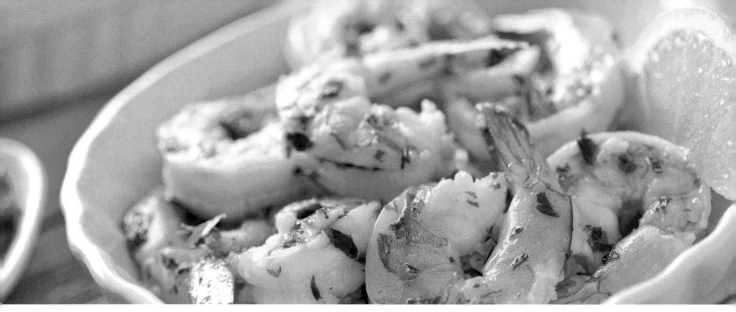

Serves: 3
Difficulty Level: 1
Cost: $$
Prep Time: 5 minutes
Cook Time: 4-5 minutes

Ingredients:

24 medium shrimp, peeled and deveined

½ cup unsalted butter

2 garlic cloves, peeled and chopped

1 Tbsp. fresh parsley, chopped

1 Tbsp. freshly squeezed lemon juice

Nutrition Facts
(Per Serving)

Calories: 485
Carbs: 4g
Fiber: 0g
Net Carbs: 4g
Protein: 41g
Fat: 34g

% calories from
Fat 63%
Carbs 3%
Protein 34%

GARLIC BUTTERED SHRIMP

Directions:

1. Start by heating a large skillet over low-medium heat with the butter.

2. Add the shrimp and cook for about 4-5 minutes or until pink.

3. During the last minute of cooking time, add in the garlic.

4. Transfer to a serving bowl and drizzle with lemon juice and garnish with fresh parsley.

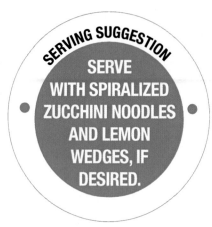

SERVING SUGGESTION

SERVE WITH SPIRALIZED ZUCCHINI NOODLES AND LEMON WEDGES, IF DESIRED.

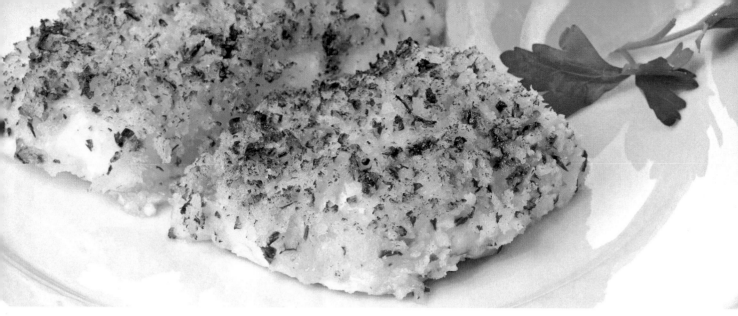

Serves: 2
Difficulty Level: 2
Cost: $$
Prep Time: 10 minutes
Cook Time: 12-15 minutes

Ingredients:

2 cod fillets

½ cup almond flour

¼ cup freshly chopped parsley

1 tsp. garlic powder

1 tsp. onion powder

Salt & pepper to taste

1 Tbsp. freshly squeezed lemon juice

SERVING SUGGESTION

SERVE WITH FRESH PARSLEY AND LEMON WEDGES, IF DESIRED.

ALMOND-CRUSTED COD

GF **DF** **P**

Directions:

1. Start by preheating the oven to 400°F and greasing a baking dish.

2. Add the almond flour, parsley, garlic powder, onion, powder, salt and pepper to a large mixing bowl.

3. Press each fillet into the almond flour mixture and then place into the baking dish.

4. Bake for 12-15 minutes or until the fish is cooked through and firm.

5. Drizzle with lemon juice.

Nutrition Facts (Per Serving)
Calories: 138   Carbs: 4g   Fiber: 1g   Net Carbs: 3g
Protein: 22g   Fat: 4g
% calories from   Fat 26%   Carbs 11%   Protein 63%

LEMON ROSEMARY SHRIMP GF P DF

Serves: 3
Difficulty Level: 1
Cost: $$
Prep Time: 5 minutes
Cook Time: 6-9 minutes

SERVING SUGGESTION

SERVE WITH A SIDE SALAD AND LEMON WEDGES, IF DESIRED.

Ingredients:

24 jumbo shrimp, peeled and deveined (tail left on)

2 Tbsp. olive oil

1 garlic clove, peeled and chopped

1 Tbsp. freshly chopped rosemary

1 Tbsp. freshly squeezed lemon juice

Salt & pepper to taste

Directions:

1. Start by heating a large skillet over low-medium heat with the olive oil.

2. Add the shrimp and cook for about 4-5 minutes or until pink.

3. Add in the garlic, rosemary and lemon juice, and stir.

4. Transfer to a serving bowl and enjoy.

Nutrition Facts (Per Serving)

Calories: 295
Carbs: 4g
Fiber: 1g
Net Carbs: 3g
Protein: 40g
Fat: 13g

% calories from
Fat 40%
Carbs 5%
Protein 55%

LEMON CILANTRO BAKED TILAPIA WITH BROCCOLI (GF) (P) (DF)

Serves: 2   Difficulty Level: 2

Cost: $$ Prep Time: 10 minutes   Cook Time: 20 minutes

Ingredients:

2 tilapia fillets

2 Tbsp. olive oil

2 Tbsp. freshly squeezed lemon juice

1 cup broccoli florets

1 Tbsp. freshly chopped cilantro

Salt & pepper to taste

SERVING SUGGESTION

SERVE WITH EXTRA LEMON JUICE OR LEMON WEDGES, IF DESIRED.

Directions:

1. Start by preheating the oven to 425°F and greasing a baking dish.

2. Season the tilapia with the olive oil, cilantro, lemon juice, salt and pepper.

3. Bake for 20 minutes or until the fish begins to flake, turning halfway through.

4. While the tilapia is cooking, steam or boil the broccoli until tender.

5. Serve the tilapia with the broccoli.

Nutrition Facts (Per Serving)

Calories: 239   Carbs: 3g   Fiber: 1g   Net Carbs: 2g
Protein: 22g   Fat: 16g

% calories from   Fat 59%   Carbs 5%   Protein 36%

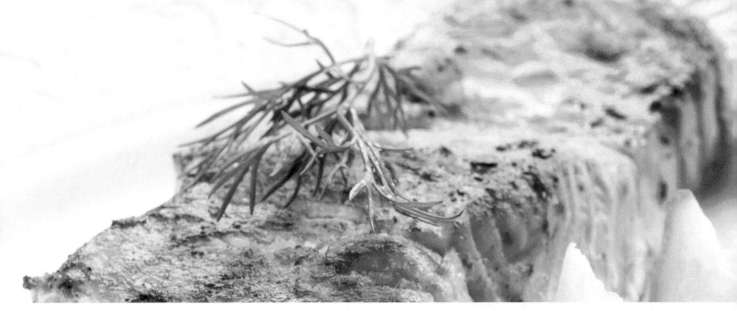

Serves: 2
Difficulty Level: 2
Cost: $$
Prep Time: 10 minutes
Cook Time: 12-15 minutes

Ingredients:

2 large salmon fillets

2 Tbsp. olive oil

½ tsp. salt

½ tsp. black pepper

1 Tbsp. freshly squeezed lemon juice

Sliced lemon for garnish

Fresh dill for garnish

Nutrition Facts
(Per Serving)

Calories: 359
Carbs: 1g
Fiber: 0g
Net Carbs: 1g
Protein: 35g
Fat: 25g

% calories from
Fat 61%
Carbs 1%
Protein 38%

BAKED LEMON SALMON

GF DF P

Directions:

1. Start by preheating the oven to 400°F and coating a baking dish with oil.

2. Add the salmon to the dish and season with the olive oil, salt, pepper and lemon juice.

3. Bake for 12-15 minutes or until the fish begins to flake.

4. Garnish with sliced lemon and fresh dill.

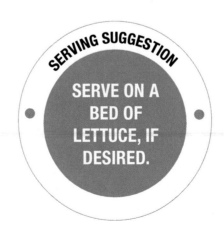

SERVING SUGGESTION

SERVE ON A BED OF LETTUCE, IF DESIRED.

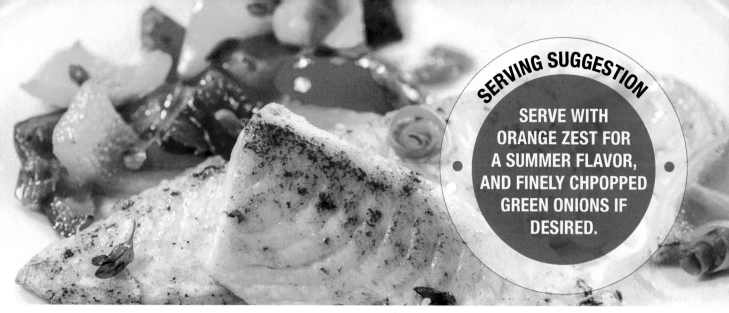

Serves: 2
Difficulty Level: 2
Cost: $$
Prep Time: 10 minutes
Cook Time: 30 minutes

Ingredients:

2 tilapia fillets

1 Tbsp. freshly squeezed lemon juice

1 garlic clove, peeled and chopped

1 tsp. freshly chopped parsley

1 red bell pepper, cored and chopped

1 yellow bell pepper, cored and chopped

4 Tbsp. olive oil

Salt & pepper to taste

TILAPIA WITH SUMMER (GF) (DF) (P) VEGETABLES

Directions:

1. Start by preheating the oven to 375°F and coating a baking dish with 1 tablespoon of olive oil.

2. Next, rinse the tilapia fillets and pat dry. Add to the baking dish.

3. Season with the garlic, parsley, salt, pepper and 2 tablespoons of olive oil. Bake for about 30 minutes or until the fish begins to flake.

4. While the tilapia is cooking, chop the peppers and sauté them in 1 tablespoon of olive oil until tender.

Nutrition Facts (Per Serving)
Calories: 322   Carbs: 10g   Fiber: 2g   Net Carbs: 8g
Protein: 22g   Fat: 23g
% calories from   Fat 62%   Carbs 12%   Protein 26%

VEGETABLE COD SOUP

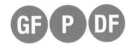

Serves: 6
Difficulty Level: 2
Cost: $$
Prep Time: 10 minutes
Cook Time: 15-17 minutes

Ingredients:

4 cod fillets, skin removed

4 cups reduced-sodium vegetable broth

2 carrots, peeled and chopped

1 yellow onion, peeled and chopped

2 garlic cloves, peeled and chopped

1 Tbsp. Italian seasoning

Salt & pepper to taste

Nutrition Facts
(Per Serving)

Calories: 150
Carbs: 14g
Fiber: 2g
Net Carbs: 12g
Protein: 10g
Fat: 6g

% calories from
Fat 36%   Carbs 37%   Protein 27%

Directions:

1. Start by cutting the cod into 1-inch pieces and set aside.

2. Add all of the ingredients, minus the fish, to a large stockpot and bring to a boil. Simmer for 10 minutes.

3. Add the cod and boil for another 5-7 minutes or until the fish begins to flake with a fork.

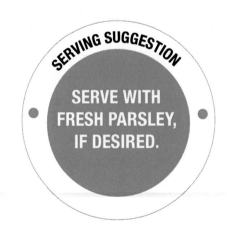

SERVING SUGGESTION
SERVE WITH FRESH PARSLEY, IF DESIRED.

"NOODLES" WITH GARLIC SHRIMP & TOMATOES GF DF P

Serves: 2
Difficulty Level: 1
Cost: $$
Prep Time: 5 minutes
Cook Time: 6-9 minutes

Ingredients:

1 large zucchini

8 shrimp, deveined

8 cherry tomatoes, halved

2 garlic cloves, peeled and chopped

2 Tbsp. olive oil

1 Tbsp. Italian seasoning

Directions:

1. Spiralize the zucchini and put to one side.

2. Start by heating a medium skillet over medium heat with the olive oil and cook the shrimp with the garlic and Italian seasoning for about 7 minutes or until the shrimp is completely pink.

3. Add the zucchini and tomatoes to the pan for about 5 minutes for 'al dente' noodles (cook for 1-2 minutes longer for softer noodles).

4. Serve whilst warm and enjoy.

Nutrition Facts
(Per Serving)

Calories: 272
Carbs: 8g
Fiber: 2g
Net Carbs: 6g
Protein: 22g
Fat: 18g

% calories from
Fat 57%   Carbs 11%   Protein 31%

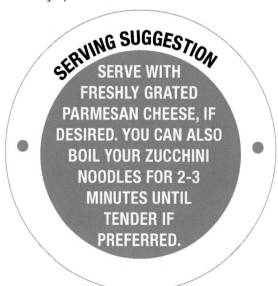

SERVING SUGGESTION

SERVE WITH FRESHLY GRATED PARMESAN CHEESE, IF DESIRED. YOU CAN ALSO BOIL YOUR ZUCCHINI NOODLES FOR 2-3 MINUTES UNTIL TENDER IF PREFERRED.

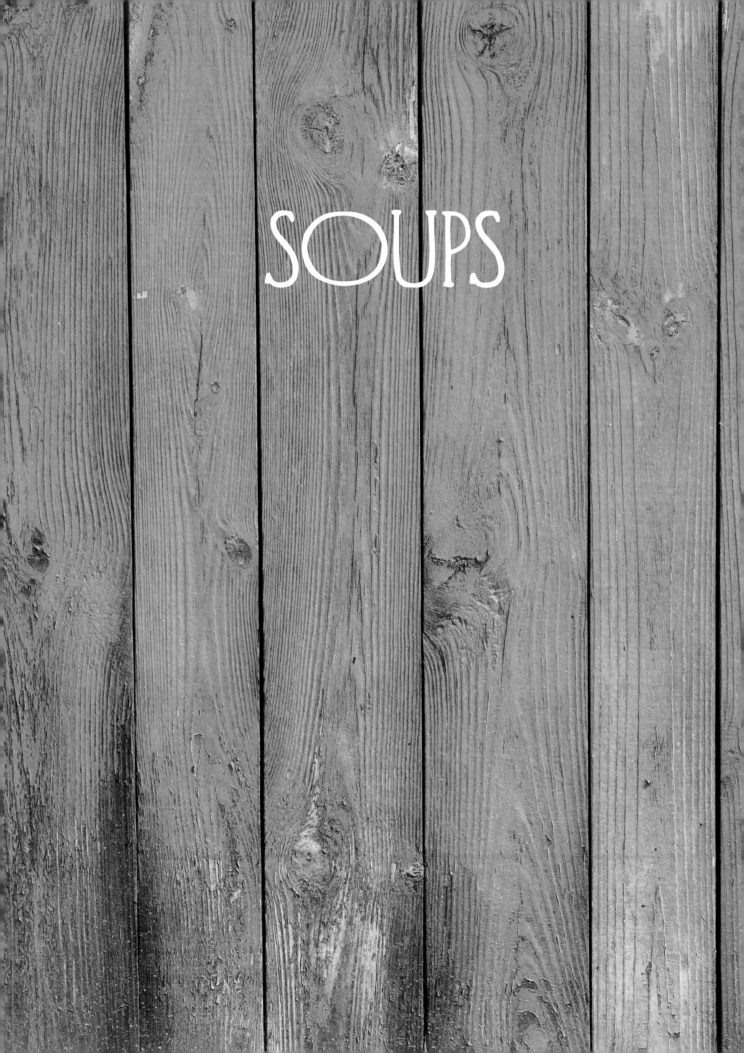
SOUPS

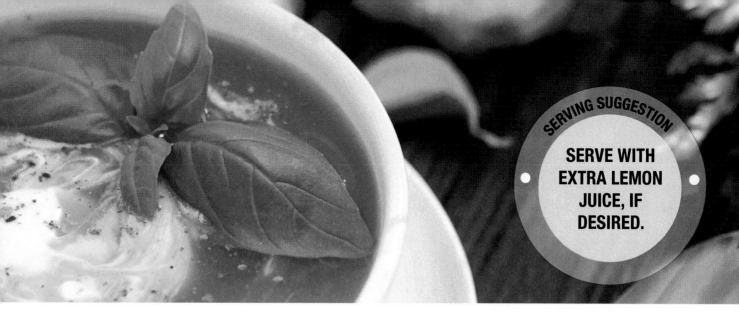

SERVING SUGGESTION

SERVE WITH EXTRA LEMON JUICE, IF DESIRED.

Serves: 4
Difficulty Level: 1
Cost: $$
Prep Time: 5 minutes
Cook Time: 15 minutes

Ingredients:

1 cup diced tomatoes

4 cups reduced-sodium vegetable broth

½ cup full-fat coconut milk

1 red onion, peeled and sliced

2 garlic cloves, peeled and chopped

1 red bell pepper, cored, seeded and chopped

Salt & pepper to taste

Fresh basil for serving

CREAMY (GF) (V) (DF) (P) MEDITERRANEAN TOMATO SOUP

Directions:

1. Start by heating a large stockpot over medium heat and add all of the ingredients, minus the coconut milk, into the pot. Bring to a boil.

2. Simmer for 15 minutes, add the coconut milk, and stir.

3. Using an immersion blender, blend the soup until smooth.

4. Serve with fresh basil.

Nutrition Facts
(Per Serving)

Calories: 138
Carbs: 9g
Fiber: 2g
Net Carbs: 7g
Protein: 7g
Fat: 9g

% calories from
Fat 56%   Carbs 25%   Protein 19%

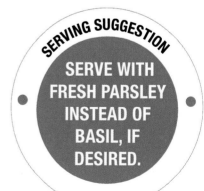

SERVING SUGGESTION

SERVE WITH FRESH PARSLEY INSTEAD OF BASIL, IF DESIRED.

MUSHROOM & COCONUT SOUP

Serves: 4
Difficulty Level: 1
Cost: $$
Prep Time: 5 minutes
Cook Time: 20-25 minutes

GF V DF P

SERVING SUGGESTION

SERVE WITH FRESH SPINACH INSTEAD OF THE COLLARD GREENS, IF DESIRED.

Ingredients:

1 cup button mushrooms, halved

3 cups reduced-sodium vegetable broth

1 cup full-fat coconut milk

2 shallots, peeled and chopped

1 cup collard greens, chopped

1 tsp. crushed red pepper

2 garlic cloves, peeled and chopped

1 tsp. dried thyme

1 tsp. dried oregano

Salt & pepper to taste

Directions:

1. Start by heating a large stockpot over medium to high heat and adding all of the ingredients. Bring to a boil.

2. Simmer for 20-25 minutes.

3. Enjoy.

Nutrition Facts (Per Serving)
Calories: 194
Carbs: 10g
Fiber: 2g
Net Carbs: 8g
Protein: 7g
Fat: 16g

% calories from
Fat 68%
Carbs 19%
Protein 13%

SAUSAGE & KALE TUSCAN SOUP GF

Serves: 6   Difficulty Level: 1
Cost: $$ Prep Time: 5 minutes
Cook Time: 20 minutes

SERVING SUGGESTION

SERVE WITH FRESHLY GRATED PARMESAN CHEESE, IF DESIRED

Ingredients:

1 lb. cooked turkey sausage, sliced

6 cups reduced-sodium chicken broth

½ cup heavy cream (use full-fat unsweetened coconut milk for a Paleo version)

2 cups kale, chopped

1 Tbsp. capers

1 red onion, peeled and sliced

2 garlic cloves, peeled and chopped

½ tsp. paprika

Salt & pepper to taste

Directions:

1. Start by heating a large stockpot over medium heat and adding all of the ingredients, minus the heavy cream, into the pot. Bring to a boil.

2. Simmer for 15 minutes, add the heavy cream; and stir.

3. Simmer for another 5 minutes and then enjoy.

Nutrition Facts (Per Serving)
Calories: 350   Carbs: 6g   Fiber: 1g   Net Carbs: 5g
Protein: 21g   Fat: 27g

% calories from   Fat 69%   Carbs 7%   Protein 24%

CREAMY CAULIFLOWER SOUP

GF **V**

Serves: 4
Difficulty Level: 1
Cost: $$
Prep Time: 5 minutes
Cook Time: 15-20 minutes

SERVING SUGGESTION

GARNISH WITH EXTRA GREEN ONION, IF DESIRED.

Ingredients:

1 cauliflower head, cut into florets

6 cups reduced-sodium vegetable broth

½ cup heavy cream (use full-fat coconut milk for a Paleo version)

3 green onions, chopped

2 garlic cloves, peeled and chopped

1 tsp. dried thyme

Salt & pepper to taste

Directions:

1. Start by heating a large stockpot over medium heat and adding all of the ingredients. Bring to a boil.

2. Simmer for 15-20 minutes or until the cauliflower is tender.

3. Using an immersion blender, blend the soup until smooth.

Nutrition Facts (Per Serving)

Calories: 97
Carbs: 10g
Fiber: 2g
Net Carbs: 8g
Protein: 2g
Fat: 6g

% calories from
Fat 53%
Carbs 39%
Protein 8%

FIRE-ROASTED TOMATO BASIL SOUP (GF) (DF) (V)

Serves: 4 Difficulty Level: 1
Cost: $$ Prep Time: 10 minutes
Cook Time: 20 minutes

Ingredients:

1 can (28 ounces) fire-roasted tomatoes

1 red onion, peeled and chopped

2 garlic cloves, peeled and chopped

1 cup basil, chopped

1 cup full-fat coconut milk

¼ tsp. salt

¼ tsp. black pepper

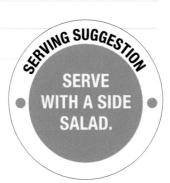

SERVING SUGGESTION
SERVE WITH A SIDE SALAD.

Directions:

1. Add all of the ingredients to a large stockpot over medium heat and bring to a boil. Simmer for 20 minutes.

2. Using an immersion blender, blend until smooth.

3. Drizzle with extra coconut milk, if desired.

Nutrition Facts (Per Serving)

Calories: 165 Carbs: 9g Fiber: 3g Net Carbs: 6g
Protein: 2g Fat: 14g

% calories from Fat 74% Carbs 21% Protein 2%

TUSCAN LEMON CHICKEN SOUP (GF) (DF) (P)

Serves: 4
Difficulty Level: 1
Cost: $$
Prep Time: 10 minutes
Cook Time: 15-20 minutes

SERVING SUGGESTION

SERVE WITH EXTRA LEMON JUICE, IF DESIRED.

Ingredients:

1 cup cooked rotisserie-style chicken, torn into bite-sized pieces

6 cups reduced-sodium chicken broth

Juice from 1 lemon

2 carrots, peeled and chopped

1 red onion, peeled and chopped

2 garlic cloves, peeled and chopped

1 tsp. fresh thyme

1 Tbsp. fresh parsley

Salt & pepper to taste

Directions:

1. Start by heating a large stockpot over medium to high heat and adding all of the ingredients, minus the fresh parsley. Stir and bring to a boil.

2. Simmer for 15-20 minutes or until the carrots are tender.

3. Serve with fresh parsley.

Nutrition Facts (Per Serving)
Calories: 140
Carbs: 9g
Fiber: 2g
Net Carbs: 7g
Protein: 18g
Fat: 3g

% calories from
Fat 20%
Carbs 27%
Protein 53%

CAULIFLOWER & CAPER SOUP

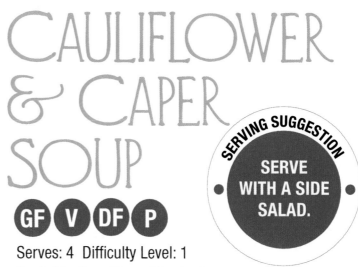

SERVING SUGGESTION
SERVE WITH A SIDE SALAD.

GF V DF P

Serves: 4   Difficulty Level: 1
Cost: $$ Prep Time: 10 minutes
Cook Time: 20-25 minutes

Ingredients:

6 cups reduced-sodium vegetable broth

1 cauliflower head, cut into florets

¼ cup capers

1 red onion, peeled and chopped

2 garlic cloves, peeled and chopped

1 Tbsp. olive oil

Salt & pepper to taste

Directions:

1. Start by heating a large stockpot over medium heat with all of the ingredients, minus the olive oil.

2. Bring the soup to a boil and simmer for 15-20 minutes or until the cauliflower is tender.

3. Using an immersion blender, blend the soup until smooth.

4. Drizzle with olive oil and enjoy.

Nutrition Facts (Per Serving)
Calories: 119   Carbs: 8g   Fiber: 3g   Net Carbs: 5g
Protein: 9g   Fat: 6g
% calories from   Fat 44%   Carbs 26%   Protein 30%

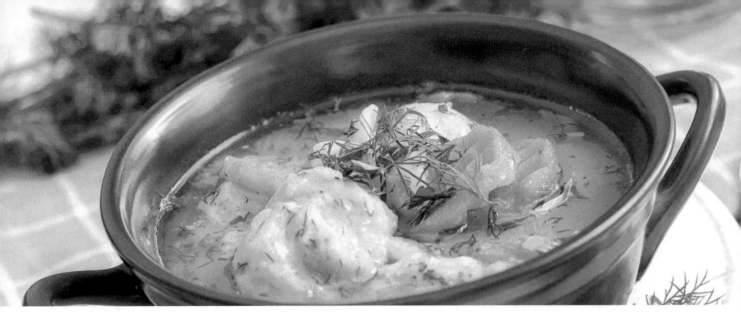

Serves: 6
Difficulty Level: 1
Cost: $$
Prep Time: 15 minutes
Cook Time: 25 minutes

Ingredients:

1 lb. boneless and skinless chicken breasts, cubed

6 cups reduced-sodium chicken broth

2 carrots, peeled and chopped

¼ cup pitted Greek olives

2 Tbsp. capers

1 red onion, peeled and sliced

2 garlic cloves, peeled and chopped

1 tsp. dried oregano

1 tsp. fresh dill

Salt & pepper to taste

1 Tbsp. olive oil for cooking

MEDITERRANEAN -STYLE CHICKEN SOUP GF DF P

Directions:

1. Start by heating a large stockpot over medium heat with the olive oil. Add the chicken and cook until the center is no longer pink.

2. Add the remaining ingredients and stir to combine. Bring to a boil and simmer for 15-20 minutes.

Nutrition Facts
(Per Serving)

Calories: 92
Carbs: 6g
Fiber: 1g
Net Carbs: 5g
Protein: 10g
Fat: 3g

% calories from
Fat 30%
Carbs 26%
Protein 44%

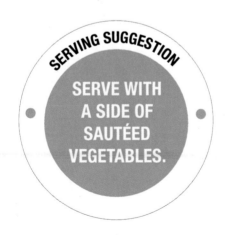

SERVING SUGGESTION

SERVE WITH A SIDE OF SAUTÉED VEGETABLES.

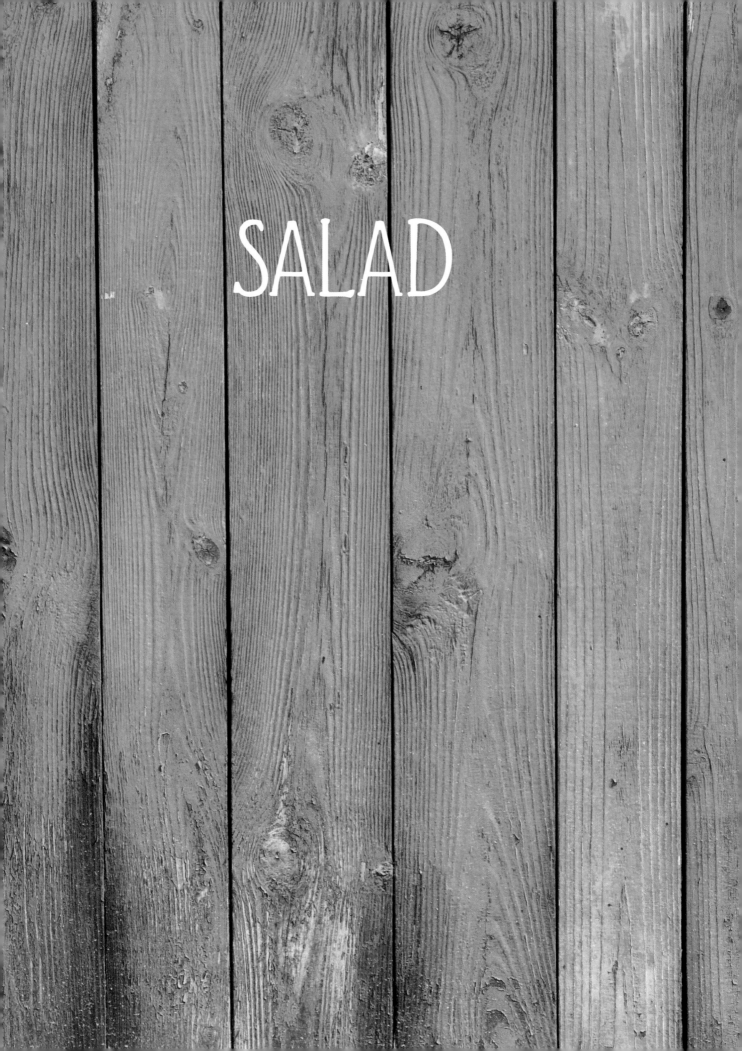

SALAD

GREEK SALAD GF V

Serves: 2
Difficulty Level: 1
Cost: $$
Prep Time: 10 minutes +
30 minutes of chilling time
Cook Time: 0 minutes

SERVING SUGGESTION

SERVE AS A REFRESHING SNACK OR SIDE SALAD.

Ingredients:

1 tomato, chopped

1 cucumber, chopped

1 red onion, peeled and sliced

¼ cup black pitted olives

¼ cup cubed feta cheese (eliminate for a Paleo version)

1 Tbsp. olive oil

1 handful fresh parsley

Salt & pepper to taste

Directions:

1. Place all ingredients, minus the olive oil, salt and pepper, into a large mixing bowl and toss to combine.

2. Drizzle with olive oil and season with salt and pepper.

3. Chill for 30 minutes before serving, if desired.

Nutrition Facts (Per Serving)

Calories: 161
Carbs: 9g
Fiber: 3g
Net Carbs: 6g
Protein: 4g
Fat: 13g

% calories from
Fat 69%
Carbs 21%
Protein 10%

LIGHT SALMON SALAD

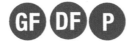

Serves: 1   Difficulty Level: 1
Cost: $$ Prep Time: 10 minutes
Cook Time: 0 minutes

Ingredients:

3 ounces of canned salmon, drained

1 cup arugula

1 cup spinach

1 radish, sliced

8 baby tomatoes, sliced

1 Tbsp. olive oil

Salt & pepper to taste

Directions:

1. Place all of the ingredients into a mixing bowl and gently toss.

2. Transfer to a serving plate and enjoy.

Nutrition Facts
(Per Serving)
Calories: 256
Carbs: 4g
Fiber: 2g
Net Carbs: 2g
Protein: 19g
Fat: 20g

% calories from
Fat 66%
Carbs 6%
Protein 28%

SERVING SUGGESTION

SERVE WITH CANNED TUNA INSTEAD OF SALMON, IF DESIRED.

ZESTY SUMMER-STYLE TUNA SALAD GF DF P

Serves: 2
Difficulty Level: 1
Cost: $
Prep Time: 10 minutes
Cook Time: 0 minutes

SERVING SUGGESTION

SERVE ALONE OR WITH FRESHLY SLICED VEGETABLES.

Ingredients:

1 can (5 ounces) tuna, drained

1 cucumber, chopped

1 yellow bell pepper, chopped

½ red bell pepper, chopped

2 Tbsp. freshly squeezed lemon juice

Salt & pepper to taste

Fresh cilantro for serving

Directions:

1. Place all ingredients in a mixing bowl and stir to combine.

2. Top with fresh cilantro and enjoy.

Nutrition Facts (Per Serving)
Calories: 220
Carbs: 13g
Fiber: 2g
Net Carbs: 11g
Protein: 26g
Fat: 8g

% calories from
Fat 33%
Carbs 20%
Protein 47%

LEMON BEET SALAD

 GF V

Serves: 2 Difficulty Level: 1
Cost: $$ Prep Time: 10 minutes
Cook Time: 0 minutes

SERVING SUGGESTION
SERVE AS A SIDE SALAD WITH A CUP OF SOUP.

Ingredients:

2 cups fresh spinach

1 cooked beet, cubed

¼ cup cubed feta cheese(eliminate for a Paleo version)

Juice from 1 lemon

3 lemon slices, halved (for serving)

Salt & pepper to taste

Directions:

1. Assemble the salad by adding the spinach to a large plate and top with the cubed cooked beet and feta cheese. Drizzle with the fresh lemon juice.

2. Season with salt and pepper and add the sliced lemon.

Nutrition Facts
(Per Serving)
Calories: 82
Carbs: 7g
Fiber: 2g
Net Carbs: 5g
Protein: 5g
Fat: 5g

% calories from
Fat 45% Carbs 31% Protein 24%

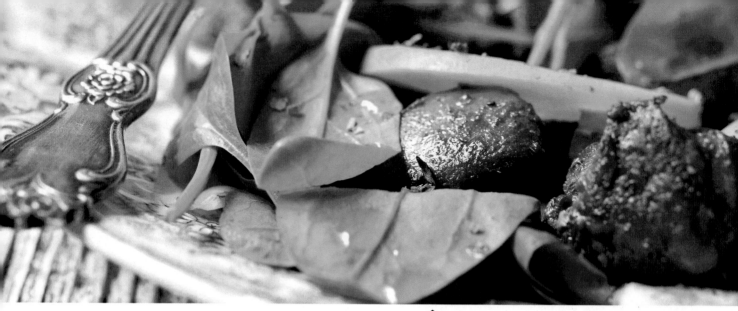

Serves: 2
Difficulty Level: 1
Cost: $$
Prep Time: 10 minutes
Cook Time: 0 minutes

Ingredients:

2 cups fresh spinach

½ cup mushrooms, sliced

½ yellow or green apple, sliced (skin left on)

2 Tbsp. olive oil

½ Tbsp. balsamic vinegar (be sure there are no added sugars or other ingredients)

1 tsp. dried oregano

Salt & pepper to taste

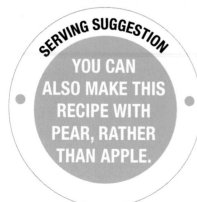

SERVING SUGGESTION

YOU CAN ALSO MAKE THIS RECIPE WITH PEAR, RATHER THAN APPLE.

SAUTÉED APPLE & MUSHROOM SALAD GF V DF P

Directions:

1. Start by heating a large skillet over medium heat with the olive oil. Add the mushrooms and apples along with the oregano. Sauté for about 5 minutes.

2. While the apples and mushrooms are cooking, add the spinach to a large plate and drizzle with the olive oil.

3. Add the cooked mushrooms and apples to the salad and season with salt and pepper.

Nutrition Facts
(Per Serving)

Calories: 164
Carbs: 11g
Fiber: 2g
Net Carbs: 9g
Protein: 2g
Fat: 15g

% calories from
Fat 74%   Carbs 23%   Protein 2%

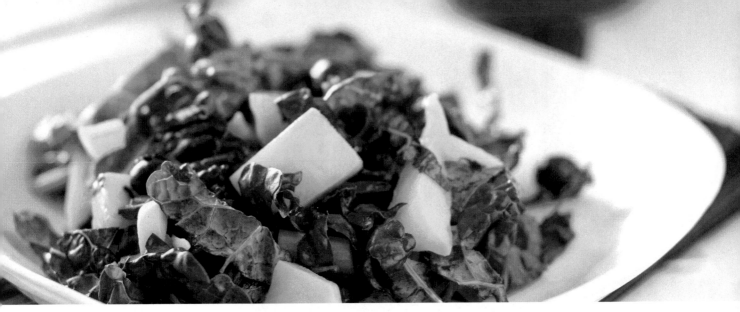

Serves: 4
Difficulty Level: 1
Cost: $$
Prep Time: 10 minutes
Cook Time: 0 minutes

MANGO & KALE SALAD

GF V DF P

Ingredients:

2 cups kale, chopped

½ cup mango, peeled and cubed

2 Tbsp. blueberries

1 Tbsp. slivered almonds

2 Tbsp. olive oil

Salt & pepper to taste

Directions:

1. Start by adding the kale to a mixing bowl with the olive oil, salt and pepper. Massage the kale and then transfer to a serving plate.

2. Top with the mango, blueberries and almonds, and enjoy.

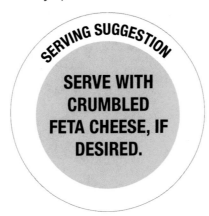

SERVING SUGGESTION

SERVE WITH CRUMBLED FETA CHEESE, IF DESIRED.

Nutrition Facts
(Per Serving)

Calories: 163
Carbs: 11g
Fiber: 1g
Net Carbs: 10g
Protein: 2g
Fat: 8g

% calories from
Fat 61%
Carbs 34%
Protein 5%

MANDARIN ORANGE & FETA SALAD GF V

Serves: 2
Difficulty Level: 1
Cost: $$
Prep Time: 10 minutes
Cook Time: 0 minutes

SERVING SUGGESTION

YOU CAN ALSO MAKE THIS SALAD USING A SPRING MIX SALAD BLEND INSTEAD OF SPINACH.

Ingredients:

2 cups fresh spinach

1 mandarin orange, peeled and sliced

¼ cup cubed feta cheese (eliminate for a Paleo version)

2 Tbsp. olive oil

½ Tbsp. balsamic vinegar

Salt & pepper to taste

Directions:

1. Start by adding the spinach, orange and feta cheese to a mixing bowl.

2. Next, drizzle with the olive oil and balsamic vinegar and season with salt and pepper and enjoy.

Nutrition Facts (Per Serving)
Calories: 212
Carbs: 10g
Fiber: 2g
Net Carbs: 8g
Protein: 4g
Fat: 18g

% calories from
Fat 74%
Carbs 18%
Protein 8%

ZESTY MEDITERRANEAN SUMMER SALAD

Serves: 2 Difficulty Level: 1
Cost: $ Prep Time: 10 minutes + 1 hour of chilling time
Cook Time: 0 minutes

Ingredients:

¼ cup sliced jalapeño pepper

½ cup crumbled feta cheese (eliminate for a Paleo version)

¼ cup canned corn, drained and rinsed (eliminate for a Paleo version)

½ cup fresh parsley, chopped

1 tomato, chopped

2 Tbsp. olive oil

1 tsp. Italian seasoning

Salt & pepper to taste

Directions:

1. Add all of the ingredients to a large mixing bowl and gently stir to combine.

2. Chill for 1 hour before serving.

Nutrition Facts
(Per Serving)
Calories: 257
Carbs: 8g
Fiber: 2g
Net Carbs: 6g
Protein: 7g
Fat: 23g

% calories from
Fat 78% Carbs 12% Protein 10%

SERVING SUGGESTION

SERVE AS A HEALTHY SNACK OR WITH A MAIN MEAL.

OLIVE &
BEET SALAD

GF **V**

Serves: 1
Difficulty Level: 1
Cost: $$
Prep Time: 10 minutes
Cook Time: 0 minutes

SERVING SUGGESTION

SERVE ALONE
OR WITH SLICED
CHEESE AND NUTS
FOR A HEALTHY
SNACK.

Ingredients:

1 cooked beet, cubed

¼ cup pitted green olives

¼ cup crumbled feta cheese (eliminate for a Paleo version)

¼ cup arugula

1 Tbsp. olive oil

Directions:

1. Place all of the ingredients into a mixing bowl and gently toss.

2. Transfer to a serving plate and enjoy.

Nutrition Facts (Per Serving)
Calories: 303
Carbs: 14g
Fiber: 3g
Net Carbs: 11g
Protein: 7g
Fat: 26g

% calories from
Fat 70%
Carbs 17%
Protein 13%

BACON & PECAN SALAD

Serves: 2   Difficulty Level: 1
Cost: $$ Prep Time: 10 minutes   Cook Time: 0 minutes

Ingredients:

2 cups spinach

1 avocado, pitted and cubed

¼ red onion, peeled and sliced

2 Tbsp. pecan halves

1 Tbsp. crumbled feta cheese (eliminate for a Paleo version)

1 Tbsp. bacon bits (be sure to use an organic nitrate free option for Paleo compliant)

1 Tbsp. olive oil

Directions:

1. Start by adding all of the ingredients, minus the olive oil, to a mixing bowl and toss to combine.

2. Drizzle with olive oil and enjoy.

Nutrition Facts
(Per Serving)
Calories: 359
Carbs: 13g
Fiber: 8g
Net Carbs: 5g
Protein: 5g
Fat: 34g

% calories from
Fat 81% Carbs 14% Protein 5%

SERVING SUGGESTION
SERVE WITH WALNUTS OR SLIVERED ALMONDS INSTEAD OF PECANS, IF DESIRED.

TOMATO & DILL EGG SALAD

Serves: 1
Difficulty Level: 1
Cost: $$
Prep Time: 10 minutes
Cook Time: 10-15 minutes

GF P

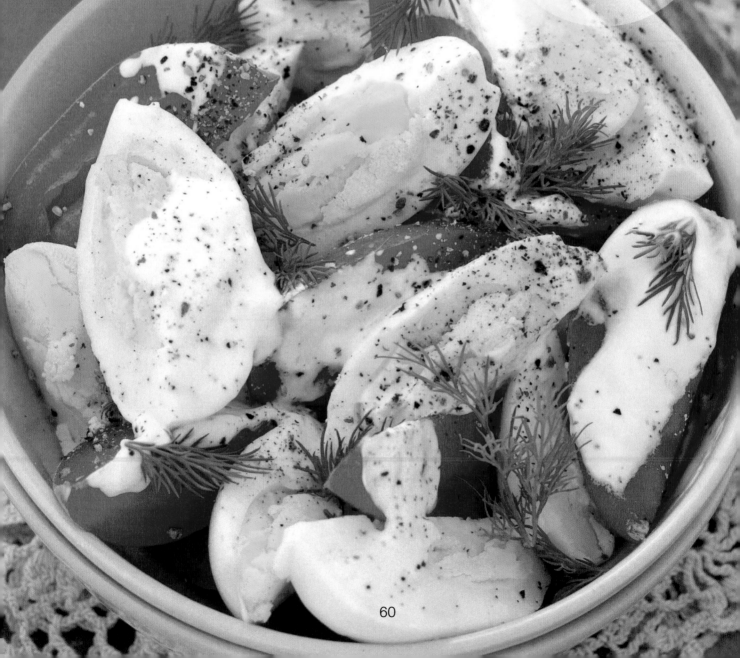

SERVING SUGGESTION

SERVE WITH
FRESH ARUGULA,
IF DESIRED.

Ingredients:

2 eggs

1 tomato, quartered

1 Tbsp. fresh dill, chopped

¼ tsp. salt

1 Tbsp. mayonnaise

Directions:

1. Start by bringing a large pot of water to a boil and boil the eggs for about 10-15 minutes or until they reach the desired tenderness. For a softer boiled egg, boil for 10 minutes.

2. While the eggs are boiling, add the tomato and dill to a mixing bowl.

3. Once cooked, allow the eggs to cool and then peel and quarter each egg. Add to the salad.

4. Season with salt and serve with mayonnaise.

Nutrition Facts (Per Serving)

Calories: 202
Carbs: 8g
Fiber: 1g
Net Carbs: 7g
Protein: 12g
Fat: 14g

% calories from
Fat 61%
Carbs 16%
Protein 23%

WATERMELON ARUGULA SALAD GF V

Serves: 1 Difficulty Level: 1
Cost: $$ Prep Time: 10 minutes Cook Time: 0 minutes

Ingredients:

2 cups arugula

½ cup watermelon, cut into small cubes

1 Tbsp. hulled sunflower seeds

1 Tbsp. crumbled feta cheese (eliminate for a Paleo version)

1 Tbsp. olive oil

Directions:

1. Start by adding all of the ingredients, minus the olive oil, to a mixing bowl and toss to combine.

2. Drizzle with olive oil and enjoy.

3. You can also add fresh spinach leaves or completely replace the arugula with spinach.

Nutrition Facts
(Per Serving)
Calories: 194
Carbs: 8g
Fiber: 1g
Net Carbs: 7g
Protein: 3g
Fat: 18g

% calories from
Fat 79% Carbs 16% Protein 6%

SERVING SUGGESTION

SERVE WITH BALSAMIC VINEGAR INSTEAD OF OLIVE OIL, IF DESIRED.

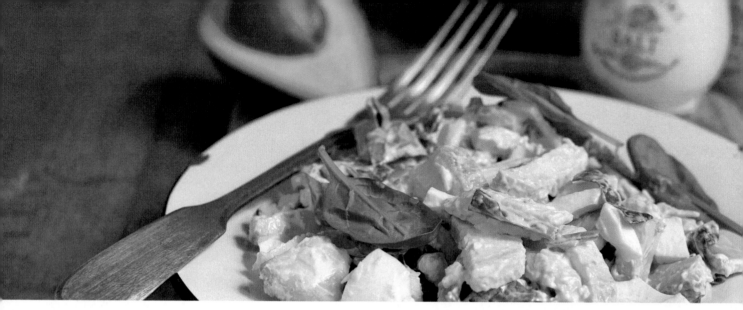

Serves: 2
Difficulty Level: 1
Cost: $$
Prep Time: 10 minutes
Cook Time: 0 minutes

Ingredients:

2 hard-boiled eggs, peeled and chopped

1 avocado, pitted and cubed

¼ cup full-fat unsweetened Greek yogurt (eliminate for a Paleo version)

1 cup fresh spinach

1 tsp. onion powder

Salt & pepper to taste

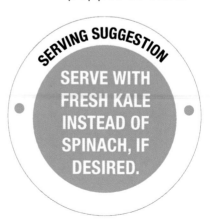

SERVING SUGGESTION

SERVE WITH FRESH KALE INSTEAD OF SPINACH, IF DESIRED.

AVOCADO & SPINACH EGG SALAD GF

Directions:

1. Start by adding the hard-boiled eggs, avocado and Greek yogurt to a mixing bowl and stir to combine.

2. Add the fresh spinach and seasoning. Stir well and enjoy.

Nutrition Facts
(Per Serving)

Calories: 297
Carbs: 12g
Fiber: 7g
Net Carbs: 5g
Protein: 11g
Fat: 25g

% calories from
Fat 71%
Carbs 15%
Protein 14%

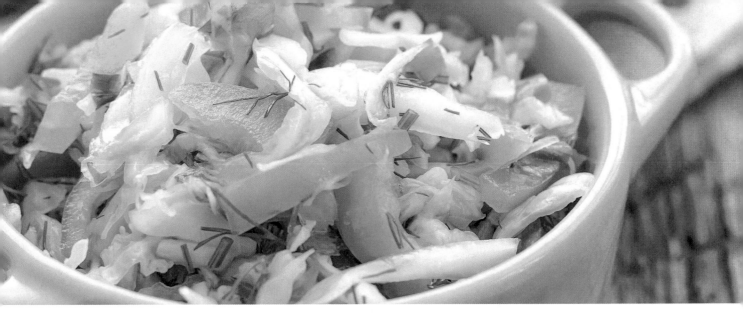

Serves: 5
Difficulty Level: 1
Cost: $$
Prep Time: 10 minutes
Cook Time: 0 minutes

Ingredients:

1 green cabbage head, chopped

1 yellow bell pepper, thinly sliced

½ cup green olives, pitted and halved

1 Tbsp. fresh dill, chopped

1 Tbsp. olive oil

Salt & pepper to taste

Nutrition Facts
(Per Serving)

Calories: 84
Carbs: 11g
Fiber: 4g
Net Carbs: 7g
Protein: 2g
Fat: 5g

% calories from
Fat 46%   Carbs 45%   Protein 8%

GREEN CABBAGE SALAD

GF V DF P

Directions:

1. Add the chopped cabbage, bell pepper and green olives to a large mixing bowl and stir gently.

2. Add in the fresh dill, drizzle with olive oil, and stir gently.

3. Season with salt and pepper and enjoy.

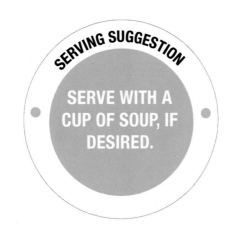

SERVING SUGGESTION

SERVE WITH A CUP OF SOUP, IF DESIRED.

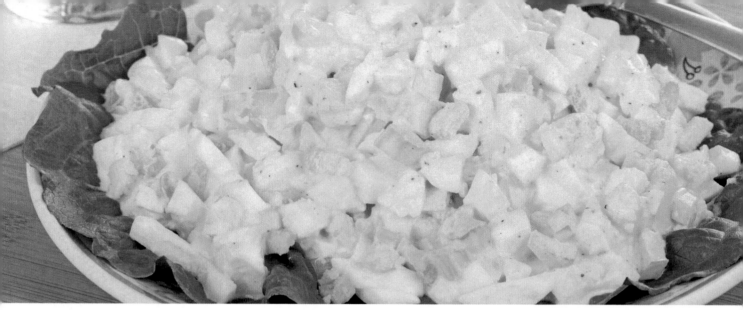

Serves: 3
Difficulty Level: 1
Cost: $$
Prep Time: 10 minutes
Cook Time: 10-15 minutes

Ingredients:

6 eggs

½ cup unsweetened full-fat Greek yogurt

1 celery stalk, chopped

½ red onion, peeled and chopped

½ tsp. salt

¼ tsp. pepper

Nutrition Facts
(Per Serving)

Calories: 160
Carbs: 4g
Fiber: 1g
Net Carbs: 3g
Protein: 18g
Fat: 10g

% calories from
Fat 51%
Carbs 9%
Protein 40%

GUILT-FREE EGG SALAD

Directions:

1. Start by bringing a large pot of water to a boil and boil the eggs for about 10-15 minutes or until they reach the desired level of cooking. If you prefer your eggs to be soft boiled, boil for 10 minutes or 15 minutes for a firmer hard-boiled egg.

2. Once cooked, allow the eggs to cool and then peel and slice in half. Add to a bowl and then mash.

3. Add the remaining ingredients and stir to combine.

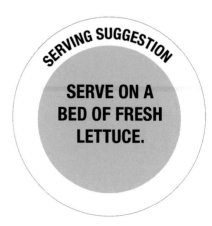

SERVING SUGGESTION

SERVE ON A BED OF FRESH LETTUCE.

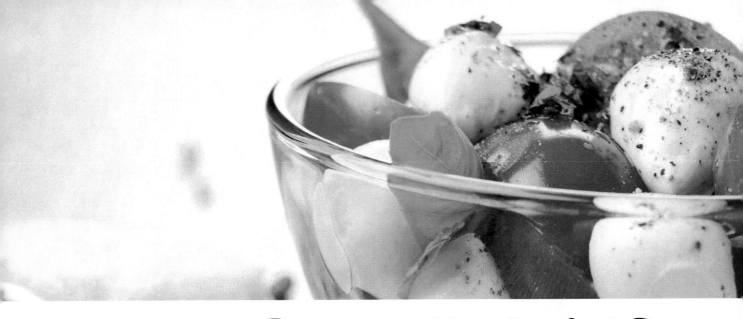

CAPRESE SALAD

GF V

Serves: 4
Difficulty Level: 1
Cost: $$
Prep Time: **10 minutes + 1 hour of chilling time**
Cook Time: 0 **minutes**

Ingredients:

12 fresh mozzarella balls

2 tomatoes, quartered

¼ cup capers

1 handful fresh basil

1 Tbsp. olive oil

½ tsp. ground black pepper

½ tsp. salt

Directions:

1. Place the mozzarella, tomatoes, capers and basil into a large mixing bowl and stir gently to combine.

2. Drizzle with olive oil and season with salt and pepper.

3. Chill for 1 hour before serving.

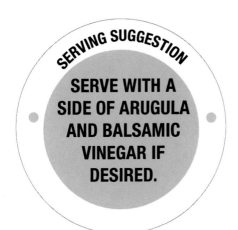

SERVING SUGGESTION

SERVE WITH A SIDE OF ARUGULA AND BALSAMIC VINEGAR IF DESIRED.

Nutrition Facts
(Per Serving)

Calories: 225
Carbs: 3g
Fiber: 1g
Net Carbs: 2g
Protein: 19g
Fat: 17g

% calories from
Fat 65%
Carbs 3%
Protein 32%

BREAKFAFST RECIPES

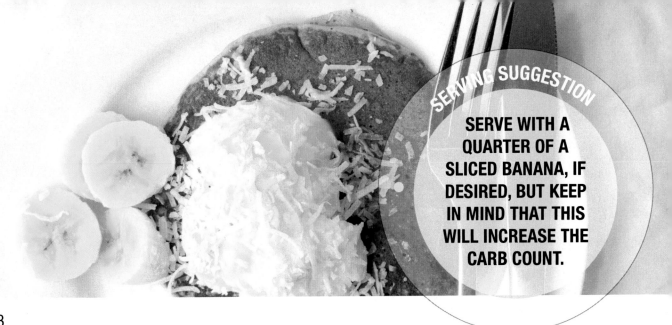

SERVING SUGGESTION

SERVE WITH A QUARTER OF A SLICED BANANA, IF DESIRED, BUT KEEP IN MIND THAT THIS WILL INCREASE THE CARB COUNT.

Serves: 3
Difficulty Level: 1
Cost: $
Prep Time: 10 minutes
Cook Time: 5 minutes

Ingredients:

1 cup full-fat unsweetened Greek yogurt (use an unsweetened coconut based yogurt for a Paleo version)

¼ cup full-fat coconut milk

¼ cup sifted coconut flour

1 egg

1 tsp. ground cinnamon

1 tsp. pure vanilla extract

1 tsp. baking powder

Coconut oil for cooking

2 Tbsp. whipped butter (for serving) (eliminate for a Paleo version)

2 Tbsp. shredded unsweetened coconut (for serving)

COCONUT & GREEK YOGURT PANCAKES GF V

Directions:

1. Start by heating a large skillet over medium heat with the coconut oil.

2. Next, add the egg, vanilla extract and coconut milk to a mixing bowl and whisk.

3. Add in the remaining ingredients (except whipped butter and shredded coconut) and whisk to combine.

4. Pour ¼ cup of the batter into the preheated pan at a time and cook for about 1 minute on each side.

5. Serve with the butter and shredded coconut.

Nutrition Facts (Per Serving)
Calories: 288   Carbs: 18g   Fiber: 9g   Net Carbs: 9g
Protein: 14g Fat: 18g

% calories from
Fat 56%   Carbs 25%   Protein 19%

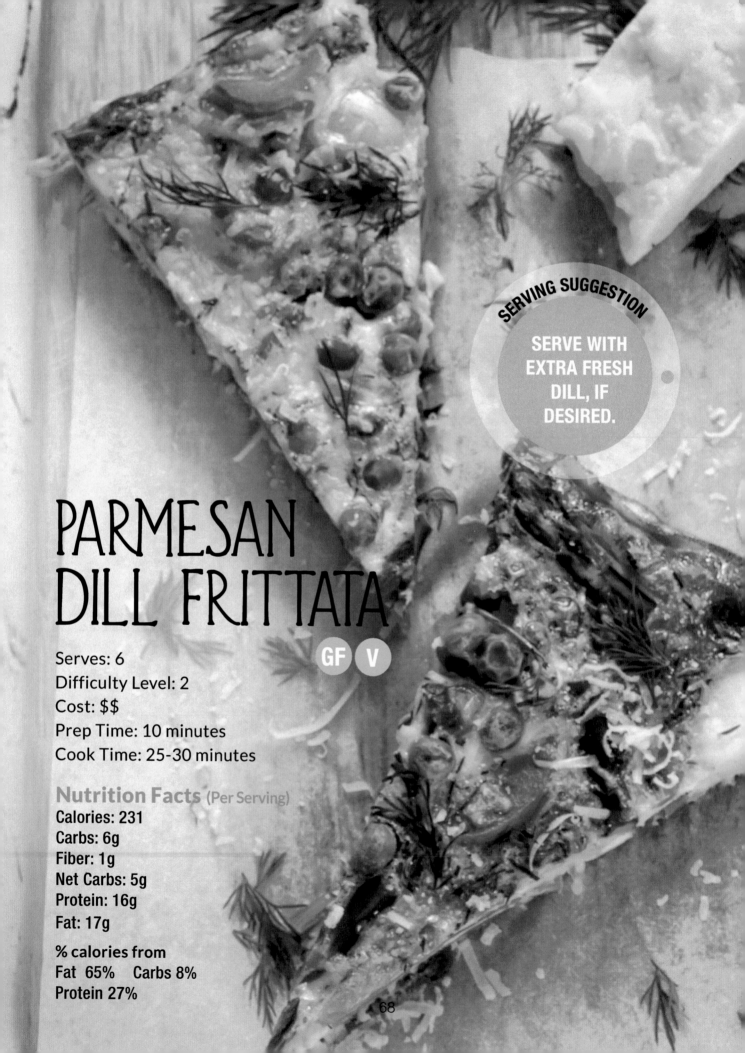

SERVING SUGGESTION

SERVE WITH EXTRA FRESH DILL, IF DESIRED.

PARMESAN DILL FRITTATA

GF V

Serves: 6
Difficulty Level: 2
Cost: $$
Prep Time: 10 minutes
Cook Time: 25-30 minutes

Nutrition Facts (Per Serving)

Calories: 231
Carbs: 6g
Fiber: 1g
Net Carbs: 5g
Protein: 16g
Fat: 17g

% calories from
Fat 65%   Carbs 8%
Protein 27%

Ingredients:

12 eggs

¼ cup unsweetened almond milk

¼ cup grated Parmesan cheese (eliminate for a Paleo version)

¼ cup frozen peas

2 carrots, peeled and chopped

1 red onion, peeled and chopped

¼ cup scallions, chopped

1 Tbsp. fresh dill

2 Tbsp. olive oil

Salt & pepper taste

Directions:

1. Start by preheating the oven to 425°F and heating a large cast-iron skillet over medium heat on the stove with the olive oil.

2. Add the carrots, onions, scallions and peas. Cook for about 1 minute.

3. While the vegetables are cooking, add the eggs, Parmesan cheese, dill and milk to a large mixing bowl and whisk.

4. Pour the egg mixture into the skillet over the vegetables, and cook for 2 minutes.

5. Next, place the skillet in the oven, and cook for 20-30 minutes or until the mixture is set in the center.

6. Season with salt and pepper.

7. Slice into 6 servings and enjoy.

VANILLA & BLACKBERY BREAKFAST SMOOTHIE

Serves: 2 Difficulty Level: 1 GF V
Cost: $ Prep Time: 10 minutes
Cook Time: 0 minutes

Ingredients:

1 cup unsweetened almond milk

1 cup unsweetened full-fat Greek yogurt (use an unsweetened coconut based yogurt or full-fat coconut cream for a Paleo version)

1 cup frozen blackberries

1 Tbsp. ground flaxseeds

1 tsp. pure vanilla extract

Directions:

1. Place all ingredients into a blender and blend until smooth.

2. Enjoy right away.

SERVING SUGGESTION
FOR AN EVEN MORE REFRESHING FLAVOR, ADD A TEASPOON OF PURE PEPPERMINT EXTRACT OR A HANDFUL OF FRESH MINT LEAVES.

Nutrition Facts
(Per Serving)
Calories: 151   Carbs: 13g
Fiber: 5g   Net Carbs: 8g   Protein: 12g Fat: 5g
% calories from
Fat 30%   Carbs 36%   Protein 33%

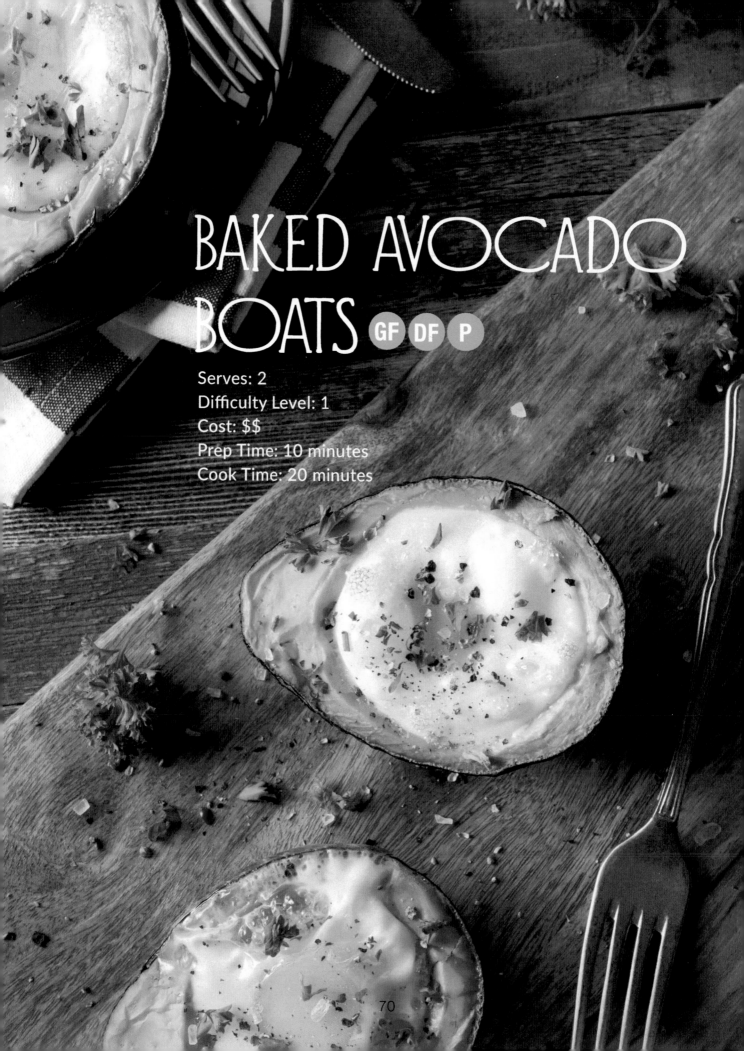

BAKED AVOCADO BOATS GF DF P

Serves: 2
Difficulty Level: 1
Cost: $$
Prep Time: 10 minutes
Cook Time: 20 minutes

Ingredients:

2 ripe avocados, pitted and halved

4 eggs

1 tsp. cracked black pepper

¼ tsp. salt

1 Tbsp. olive oil

Fresh parsley for serving

Directions:

1. Start by preheating the oven to 350°F and setting out a baking dish.

2. Next, slice the avocados in half, remove the pit, and place in the baking dish.

3. Crack the eggs into a bowl and, using a spoon, remove the yolks and place them in the center of the avocado halves. Next, spoon the egg whites into the avocado halves. Add as much as you can without any of the egg spilling out.

4. Season with salt and pepper.

5. Bake for 20 minutes or until the eggs are lightly cooked and no longer runny.

6. Once cooked, drizzle with olive oil and top with fresh parsley.

Nutrition Facts (Per Serving)

Calories: 596
Carbs: 18g
Fiber: 14g
Net Carbs: 4g
Protein: 16g
Fat: 56g

% calories from
Fat 79%
Carbs 11%
Protein 10%

SERVING SUGGESTION

SERVE WITH CRUMBLED FETA CHEESE, IF DESIRED. KEEP IN MIND THAT THIS RECIPE WOULD NO LONGER BE DAIRY-FREE IF CHEESE IS ADDED.

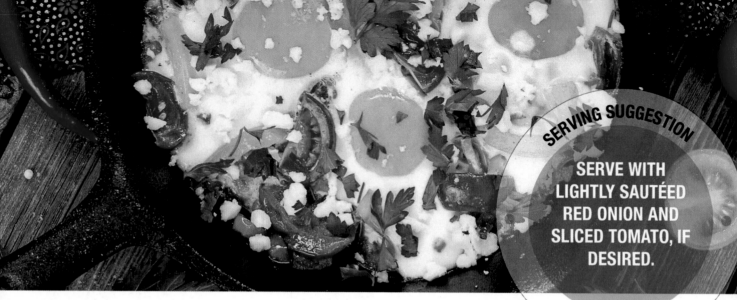

SERVING SUGGESTION

SERVE WITH LIGHTLY SAUTÉED RED ONION AND SLICED TOMATO, IF DESIRED.

Serves: 3
Difficulty Level: 2
Cost: $$
Prep Time: 10 minutes
Cook Time: 8-10 minutes

CRACKED PEPPER & FRIED EGG FRITTATA GF

Ingredients:

6 eggs

¼ cup unsweetened almond milk

1 tomato, chopped

1 jalapeño pepper, seeded and chopped

½ tsp. ground turmeric

1 Tbsp. fresh parsley

1 tsp. ground peppercorns

¼ tsp. salt

1 Tbsp. crumbled feta cheese (eliminate for a Paleo version)

Coconut oil for cooking

Directions:

1. Start by heating a large skillet over medium heat with the coconut oil.

2. Next, add three of the eggs with the unsweetened almond milk, turmeric, jalapeño pepper, tomato and ground peppercorns to a mixing bowl and whisk.

3. Pour the egg mixture into the heated skillet, and cook for about 5 minutes or until the eggs begin to set in the center.

4. Next, crack the remaining three eggs on top of the egg mixture in the pan, and cook for 3-5 minutes or until the center of the egg is lightly cooked.

5. Serve with fresh parsley, season with salt, and top with the crumbled feta cheese.

6. Slice into three servings and enjoy.

Nutrition Facts (Per Serving)

Calories: 144   Carbs: 2g   Fiber: 1g   Net Carbs: 1g   Protein: 12g   Fat: 10g
% calories from   Fat 62%   Carbs 5%   Protein 33%

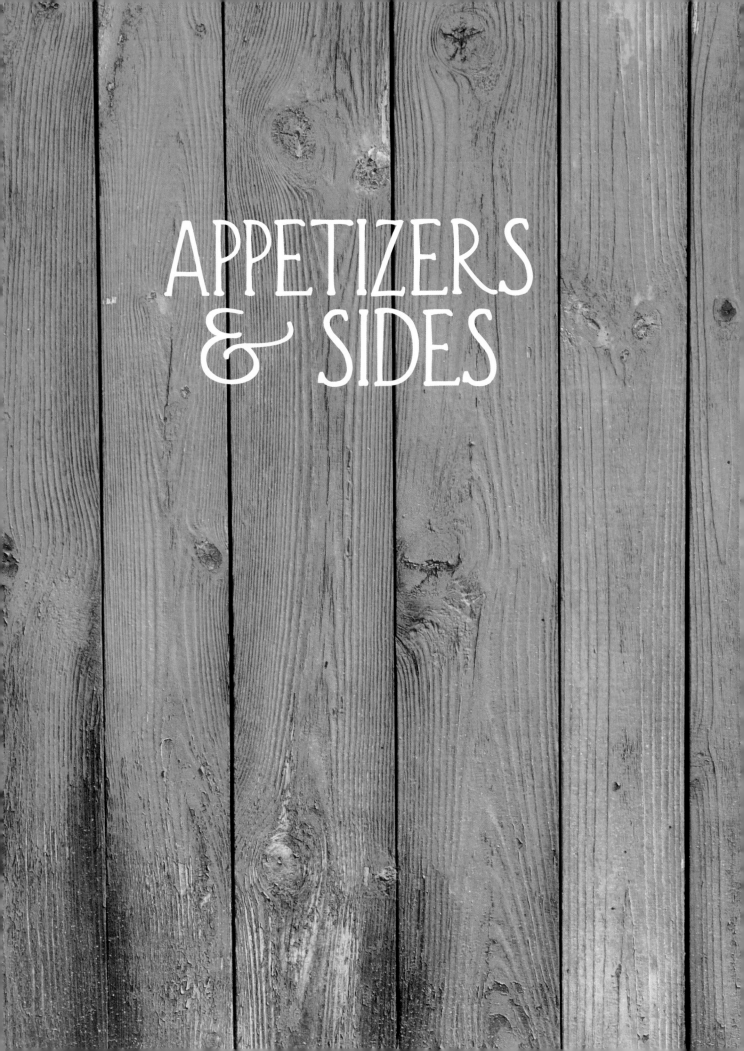

DOLMAS GF V P DF

Serves: 6
Difficulty Level: 2
Cost: $$
Prep Time: 15 minutes
Cook Time: 35 minutes

Nutrition Facts (Per Serving)
Calories: 66
Carbs: 10g
Fiber: 1g
Net Carbs: 9g
Protein: 1g
Fat: 3g

% calories from
Fat 38%
Carbs 56%
Protein 6%

SERVING SUGGESTION

SERVE WITH AN EXTRA DRIZZLE OF FRESHLY SQUEEZED LEMON JUICE, IF DESIRED.

Ingredients:

1 jar (8 ounces) grape leaves

1 garlic clove, peeled and chopped

1 yellow onion, peeled and chopped

¼ cup mushrooms, chopped

1 jalapeño pepper, chopped

¼ cup pitted olives, chopped

6 Tbsp. freshly squeezed lemon juice

1 Tbsp. fresh dill

Olive oil for cooking + 1 Tbsp. for drizzling

Salt & pepper to taste

Directions:

1. Start by heating a medium skillet over medium heat with the olive oil.

2. Chop all of the vegetables and add all of them, minus the olives, to the skillet. Sauté for 5 minutes.

3. While the vegetables are cooking, unroll the grape leaves and lay them flat on a clean and dry surface. Place 1 tablespoon of the vegetable mixture at the bottom of the leaf.

4. Drizzle the lemon juice and add the fresh dill.

5. Season with salt and pepper.

6. Start to roll the leaf by folding the bottom of the leaf up followed by folding the right and left sides in. Then, continue rolling toward the top. Do not roll the leaves too tightly.

7. After you roll the dolmas, add them to a large pot by placing them all close together. You can have two layers, if necessary.

8. Drizzle with 1 tablespoon of olive oil and add enough water to cover the dolmas. Bring to a boil and simmer for about 30 minutes.

9. Remove from the water and enjoy.

10. To store leftovers, store in a sealed container covered with water in the refrigerator.

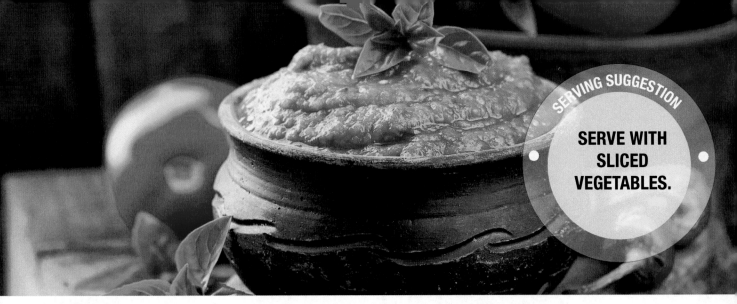

Serves: 6
Difficulty Level: 1
Cost: $
Prep Time: 5 minutes +
60 minutes of chilling time
Cook Time: 0 mins

Ingredients:

1 cup jarred roasted red peppers, drained

⅓ cup walnuts halves

1 tomato, chopped

1 jalapeño pepper, chopped

1 garlic clove, peeled and chopped

1 tsp. dried basil

1 Tbsp. olive oil

½ tsp. salt

5-MINUTE ROASTED RED PEPPER DIP (GF) (V) (DF) (P)

Directions:

1. Place all of the ingredients into a food processor and blend until smooth.

2. Chill for 1 hour before serving.

Nutrition Facts (Per Serving)

Calories: 42
Carbs: 3g
Fiber: 1g
Net Carbs: 2g
Protein: 1g
Fat: 3g

% calories from
Fat 63%
Carbs 28%
Protein 9%

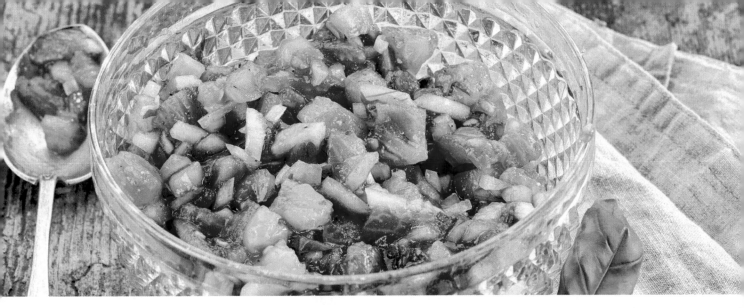

Serves: 12
Difficulty Level: 1
Cost: $
Prep Time: 65 mins
Cook Time: 0 mins

Ingredients:

2 cups tomatoes, chopped

1 red onion, peeled and chopped

¼ cup olive oil

¼ cup capers

1 Tbsp. apple cider vinegar

1 tsp. fresh thyme

1 tsp. dried oregano

½ tsp. salt

Fresh basil (for serving)

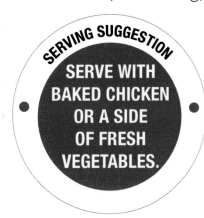

SERVING SUGGESTION
SERVE WITH BAKED CHICKEN OR A SIDE OF FRESH VEGETABLES.

MEDITERRANEAN BRUSCHETTA

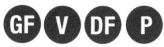

GF V DF P

Directions:

1. Start by chopping the tomatoes and onion and placing them in a large mixing bowl.

2. Add the remaining ingredients and stir to combine.

3. Chill in the refrigerator for 1 hour before serving.

4. Serve with fresh basil.

Nutrition Facts
(Per Serving)

Calories: 47
Carbs: 2g
Fiber: 1g
Net Carbs: 1g
Protein: 1g
Fat: 4g

% calories from
Fat 75%   Carbs 17%   Protein 8%

SPICED OLIVES

GF V P

Serves: 6
Difficulty Level: 1
Cost: $$
Prep Time: 10 minutes + 60 minutes, if chilling before serving
Cook Time: 0 minutes

SERVING SUGGESTION

SERVE WITH CUBED FETA CHEESE.

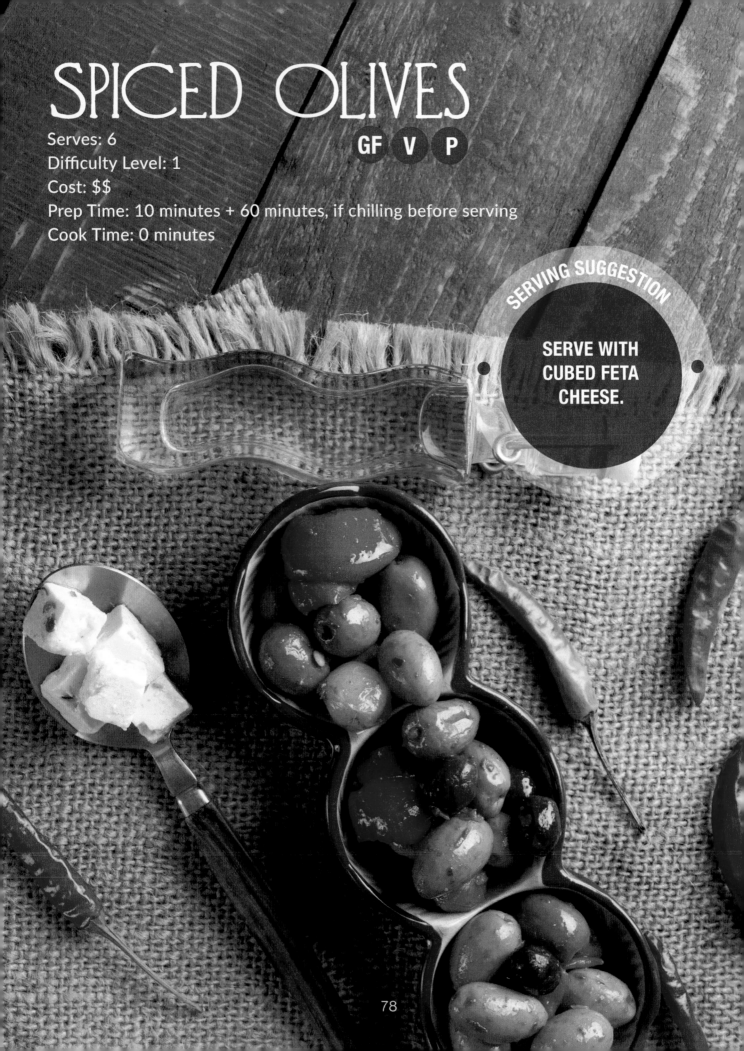

Ingredients:

1 cup mixed pitted olives

1 jalapeño pepper, chopped

¼ cup olive oil

¼ tsp. salt

⅛ tsp. cracked black pepper

Directions:

1. Add all of the ingredients to a mixing bowl and stir to combine.

2. Serve immediately or chill for an hour before serving.

Nutrition Facts (Per Serving)
Calories: 98
Carbs: 2g
Fiber: 1g
Net Carbs: 1g
Protein: 0g
Fat: 11g

% calories from
Fat 93%
Carbs 7%
Protein 0%

REFRESHING CUCUMBER SALAD GF V P

Serves: 4
Difficulty Level: 1 Cost: $
Prep Time: 10 minutes + 60 minutes of chilling time
Cook Time: 0 minutes

Ingredients:

4 cucumbers, thinly sliced

1 Tbsp. raw apple cider vinegar

1 Tbsp. freshly chopped parsley

½ tsp. salt

¼ tsp. ground peppercorns

Directions:

1. Simply place all of the ingredients into a large mixing bowl and gently toss.

2. Chill for 1 hour before serving.

Nutrition Facts
(Per Serving)
Calories: 46
Carbs: 11g
Fiber: 2g
Net Carbs: 10g
Protein: 2g
Fat: 0g

% calories from
Fat 0%
Carbs 85%
Protein 15%

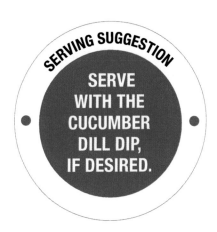

SERVING SUGGESTION

SERVE WITH THE CUCUMBER DILL DIP, IF DESIRED.

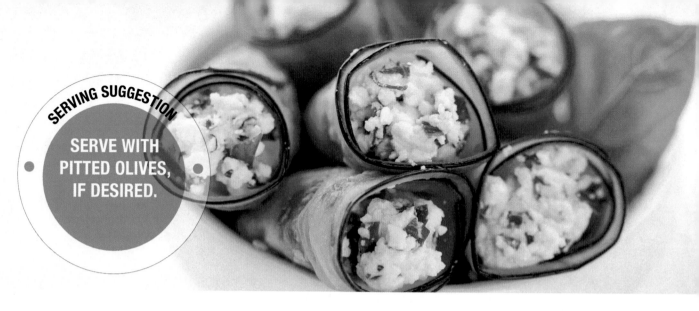

Serves: 8
Difficulty Level: 2
Cost: $
Prep Time: 25 minutes
Cook Time: 40-45 minutes

Ingredients:

1 eggplant, thinly sliced lengthwise

1 cup full-fat cottage cheese

½ cup shredded whole milk mozzarella cheese

1 egg

1 Tbsp. fresh dill

1 Tbsp. Italian seasoning

1 tsp. salt

Nutrition Facts
(Per Serving)

Calories: 47
Carbs: 4g
Fiber: 2g
Net Carbs: 2g
Protein: 4g
Fat: 2g

% calories from

Fat 36%   Carbs 32%   Protein 32%

2-CHEESE STUFFED EGG-PLANT ROLLS

Directions:

1. Start by preheating the oven to 425°F and lining a baking sheet with parchment paper.

2. Next, slice the eggplant and sprinkle with salt. Allow the eggplant to sit out for 15 minutes.

3. Next, dry the eggplant using a paper towel and place on the baking sheet. Bake for 15 minutes.

4. Allow the eggplant to cool and fill the middle of the eggplant slices with the cottage cheese, shredded mozzarella, dill and Italian seasoning. Roll up place back into the baking sheet.

5. Reduce the oven temperature to 325°F, and bake the eggplant rolls for another 25-30 minutes.

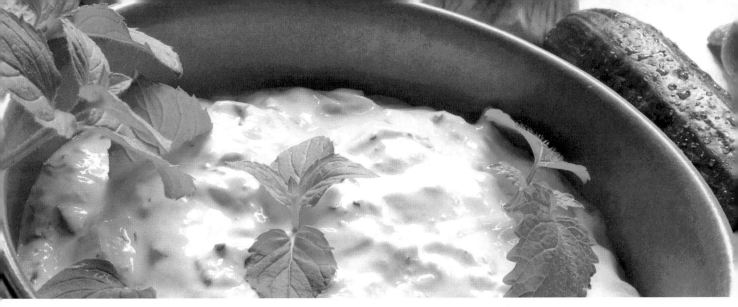

CUCUMBER & DILL DIP

GF V

Serves: 4
Difficulty Level: 1
Cost: $$
Prep Time: 10 minutes +
60 minutes of chilling time
Cook Time: 0 minutes

Ingredients:

1 cup full-fat unsweetened Greek yogurt

1 cucumber, peeled and chopped finely

1 garlic clove, peeled and chopped

2 Tbsp. fresh dill

1 Tbsp. freshly chopped mint leaves

Directions:

1. Place all ingredients into a mixing bowl and stir to combine.

2. Chill for 1 hour before serving.

Nutrition Facts
(Per Serving)

Calories: 80
Carbs: 6g
Fiber: 1g
Net Carbs: 5g
Protein: 5g
Fat: 4g

% calories from
Fat 45%
Carbs 30%
Protein 25%

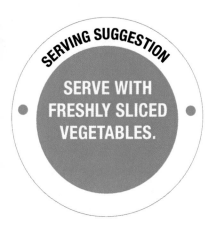

SERVING SUGGESTION

SERVE WITH FRESHLY SLICED VEGETABLES.

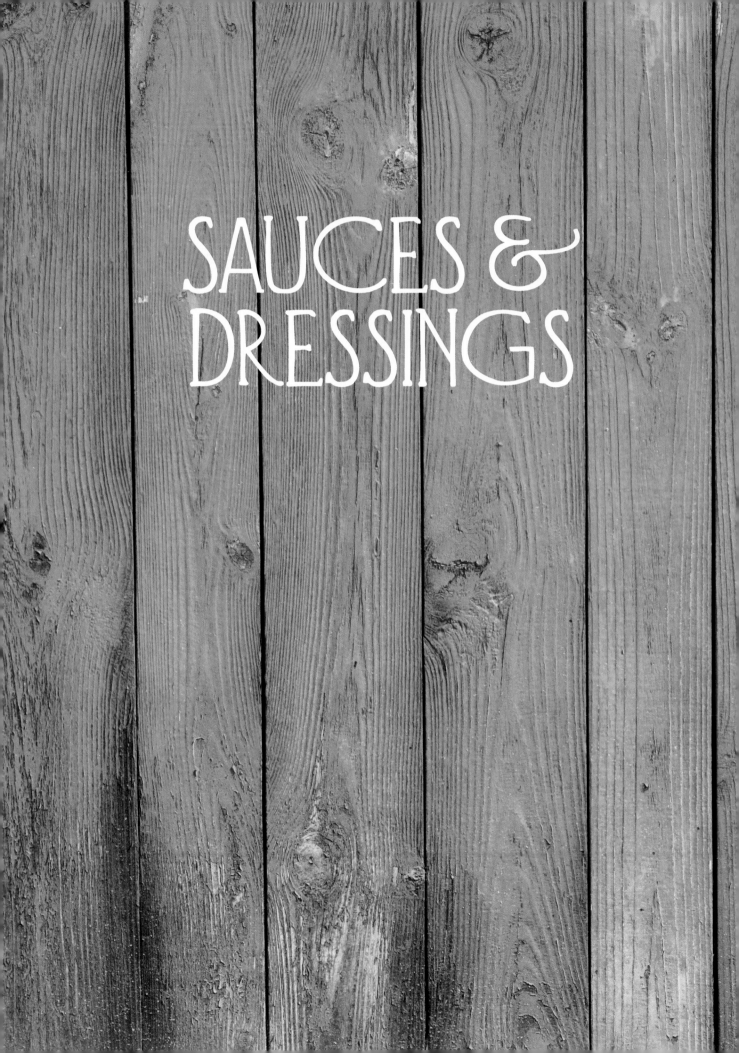

SAUCES & DRESSINGS

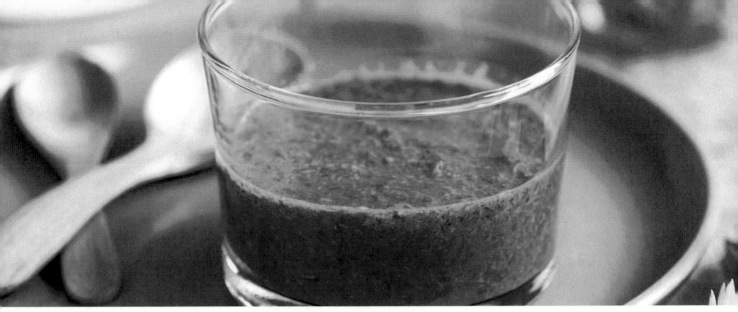

Serves: 12
Difficulty Level: 1
Cost: $$
Prep Time: 5 minutes
Cook Time: 0 minutes

Ingredients:

1 cup olive oil

2 cups fresh basil

¼ cup fresh cilantro

1 cup fresh spinach

3 garlic cloves, peeled

1 tsp. ground black pepper

1 tsp. salt

GREEN GODDESS SUPERFOOD DRESSING GF DF V P

Directions:

1. Place all of the ingredients into a blender or food processor and blend until smooth.

2. Refrigerate leftovers in the fridge.

Nutrition Facts
(Per Serving)

Calories: 147
Carbs: 1g
Fiber: 0g
Net Carbs: 1g
Protein: 0g
Fat: 17g

% calories from
Fat 97%
Carbs 3%
Protein 0%

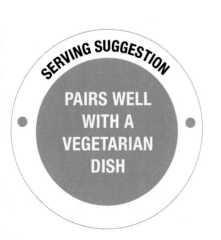

SERVING SUGGESTION

PAIRS WELL WITH A VEGETARIAN DISH

CLASSIC MEDITERRANEAN SALAD DRESSING

GF **V** **DF**

Serves: 12
Difficulty Level: 1
Cost: $
Prep Time: 5 minutes
Cook Time: 0 minutes

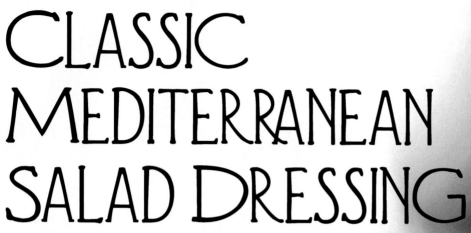

SERVING SUGGESTION

SERVE WITH SALADS OR MAKE A HEALTHY "PASTA" SALAD WITH SPIRALIZED NOODLES. PAIRS WELL WITH CHICKEN OR BEEF

Ingredients:

1 cup olive oil

¼ cup red wine vinegar

1 Tbsp. oregano

1 Tbsp. onion powder

1 Tbsp. garlic powder

1 tsp. ground black pepper

1 tsp. sea salt

Directions:

1. Place all of the ingredients into a bowl or sealed glass jar and whisk or shake the sealed jar vigorously to combine.

2. Drizzle on salads and refrigerate leftovers.

Nutrition Facts (Per Serving)

Calories: 151
Carbs: 1g
Fiber: 0g
Net Carbs: 1g
Protein: 0g
Fat: 17g

% calories from
Fat 97%
Carbs 3%
Protein 0%

LEMON & BASIL DRESSING

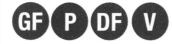

GF **P** **DF** **V**

Serves: 12 Difficulty Level: 1
Cost: $ Prep Time: 5 minutes
Cook Time: 0 minutes

Ingredients:

1 cup olive oil

Juice from 1 lemon

½ cup of freshly chopped basil

1 tsp. ground black pepper

1 tsp. sea salt

Directions:

1. Place all of the ingredients into a blender or food processor and blend until smooth.

2. Drizzle on salads and refrigerate leftovers.

Nutrition Facts

(Per Serving)

Calories: 145
Carbs: 0g
Fiber: 0g
Net Carbs: 0g
Protein: 0g
Fat: 17g

% calories from
Fat 100%
Carbs 0%
Protein 0%

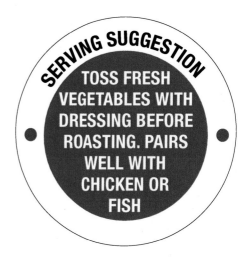

SERVING SUGGESTION

TOSS FRESH VEGETABLES WITH DRESSING BEFORE ROASTING. PAIRS WELL WITH CHICKEN OR FISH

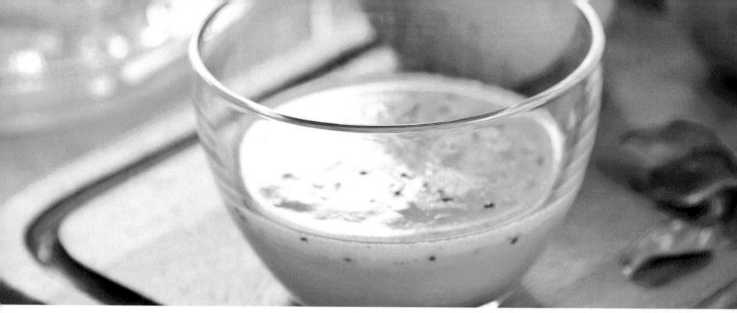

Serves: 12
Difficulty Level: 1
Cost: $
Prep Time: 5 minutes
Cook Time: 0 minutes

Ingredients:

1 cup olive oil

¼ cup freshly squeezed orange juice

¼ tsp. ground nutmeg

1 tsp. ground black pepper

1 tsp. sea salt

Nutrition Facts
(Per Serving)

Calories: 147
Carbs: 1g
Fiber: 0g
Net Carbs: 1g
Protein: 0g
Fat: 17g

% calories from
Fat 97%
Carbs 3%
Protein 0%

ORANGE & SPICE SALAD DRESSING GF DF P V

Directions:

1. Place all of the ingredients into a bowl or sealed glass jar and whisk or shake the sealed jar vigorously to combine.

2. Drizzle on salads and refrigerate leftovers.

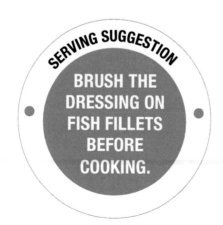

SERVING SUGGESTION

BRUSH THE DRESSING ON FISH FILLETS BEFORE COOKING.

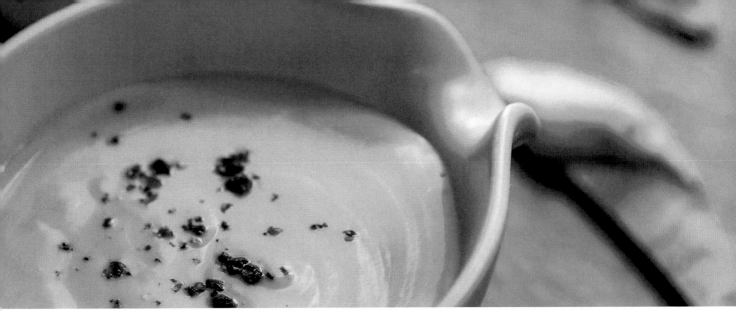

Serves: 6
Difficulty Level: 1
Cost: $$
Prep Time: 5 minutes + 1 hour of chilling time
Cook Time: 0 minutes

Ingredients:

1 cup unsweetened full-fat Greek yogurt

1 Tbsp. spicy Dijon mustard

Juice from 1 lemon

¼ tsp. paprika

1 tsp. ground black pepper

½ tsp. salt

SERVING SUGGESTION

SERVE WITH A SALAD OR AS A DIP WITH CHOPPED VEGETABLES. PAIRS WELL WITH A CHICKEN OR PORK DISH

SPICY HONEY MUSTARD DRESSING GF V

Directions:

1. Place all of the ingredients into a blender or food processor and blend until smooth.

2. Refrigerate for 1 hour before serving.

Nutrition Facts
(Per Serving)

Calories: 39
Carbs: 2g
Fiber: 0g
Net Carbs: 2g
Protein: 4g
Fat: 2g

% calories from
Fat 38%
Carbs 21%
Protein 67%

LEMON & ROSEMARY DRESSING GF V DF P

Serves: 12
Difficulty Level: 1
Cost: $
Prep Time: 5 minutes
Cook Time: 0 minutes

SERVING SUGGESTION

PAIRS WELL WITH A CHICKEN DISH

Ingredients:

1 cup olive oil

Juice from 1 lemon

1 Tbsp. fresh rosemary

1 tsp. ground black pepper

1 tsp. sea salt

Directions:

1. Place all of the ingredients into a bowl or sealed glass jar and whisk or shake the sealed jar vigorously to combine.

2. Drizzle on salads and refrigerate leftovers.

Nutrition Facts (Per Serving)

Calories: 146
Carbs: 0g
Fiber: 0g
Net Carbs: 0g
Protein: 0g
Fat: 17g

% calories from
Fat 100%
Carbs 0%
Protein 0%

LEMON & DILL DIPPING SAUCE

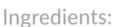

Serves: 4
Difficulty Level: 1
Cost: $
Prep Time: 5 minutes
Cook Time: 0 minutes

GF **V**

Ingredients:

1 cup unsweetened full-fat Greek yogurt

Juice from 1 lemon

1 Tbsp. fresh dill

1 tsp. ground black pepper

Directions:

1. Place all of the ingredients into a bowl and stir to combine.

2. Use as a dip for vegetables and refrigerate any leftovers.

Nutrition Facts

(Per Serving)

Calories: 58
Carbs: 3g
Fiber: 0g
Net Carbs: 3g
Protein: 5g
Fat: 3g

% calories from
Fat 46%
Carbs 20%
Protein 34%

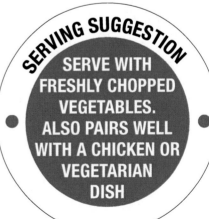

SERVING SUGGESTION
SERVE WITH FRESHLY CHOPPED VEGETABLES. ALSO PAIRS WELL WITH A CHICKEN OR VEGETARIAN DISH

AVOCADO & LIME SALAD DRESSING GF V

Serves: 6
Difficulty Level: 1
Cost: $$
Prep Time: 5 minutes + 1 hour of chilling time
Cook Time: 0 minutes

SERVING SUGGESTION

SERVE AS A DIP WITH FRESHLY CHOPPED VEGETABLES OR AS A THICK SALAD DRESSING. PAIRS WELL WITH A VEGETARIAN DISH

Ingredients:

1 cup unsweetened full-fat Greek yogurt

1 avocado, pitted and peeled

¼ cup fresh cilantro

Juice from 1 lime

1 tsp. ground black pepper

½ tsp. salt

Directions:

1. Place all of the ingredients into a blender or food processor and blend until smooth.

2. Refrigerate for 1 hour before serving.

Nutrition Facts (Per Serving)

Calories: 96
Carbs: 5g
Fiber: 2g
Net Carbs: 3g
Protein: 4g
Fat: 7g

% calories from
Fat 64%
Carbs 20%
Protein 16%

CLASSIC PESTO SAUCE

Serves: 12   Difficulty Level: 1
Cost: $$ Prep Time: 5 minutes
Cook Time: 0 minutes

(GF) (DF) (V) (P)

Ingredients:

⅔ cup olive oil

2 cups fresh basil

¼ cup pine nuts

3 garlic cloves, peeled

1 tsp. ground black pepper

1 tsp. salt

Directions:

1. Place all of the ingredients into a blender or food processor and blend until smooth.

2. Refrigerate any leftovers.

Nutrition Facts

(Per Serving)

Calories: 118
Carbs: 1g
Fiber: 0g
Net Carbs: 1g
Protein: 1g
Fat: 13g

% calories from
Fat 94%
Carbs 3%
Protein 3%

SERVING SUGGESTION

SERVE WITH SPIRALIZED ZUCCHINI FOR A HEALTHY "PASTA" DISH. ALSO PAIRS WELL WITH A CHICKEN OR BEEF DISH

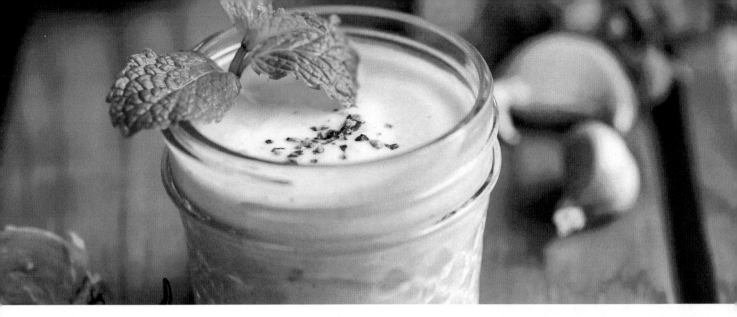

Serves: 12
Difficulty Level: 1
Cost: $$
Prep Time: 10 minutes
Cook Time: 3-5 minutes

CLASSIC TAHINI

GF **DF** **P** **V**

Ingredients:

1 cup sesame seeds

3 Tbsp. olive oil

SERVING SUGGESTION

SERVE WITH A SALAD OR AS A DIP WITH CHOPPED VEGETABLES. ALSO PAIRS WELL WITH A VEGETARIAN DISH

Directions:

1. Start by adding the sesame seeds to a large saucepan over medium heat and toast for 3-5 minutes, stirring continuously.

2. Once toasted, transfer to a large plate and allow the seeds to cool completely.

3. Add the seeds to a food processor and blend for about 1 minute or until a paste begins to form.

4. Pour in the olive oil and process for another 2 minutes or until the consistency is smooth.

5. Store in a glass jar in the refrigerator.

6. Add half a thinly sliced clove of garlic to the pan for a slight twist

Nutrition Facts
(Per Serving)

Calories: 99   Carbs: 3g   Fiber: 1g   Net Carbs: 2g
Protein: 2g   Fat: 10g

% calories from
Fat 82%   Carbs 11%   Protein 10%

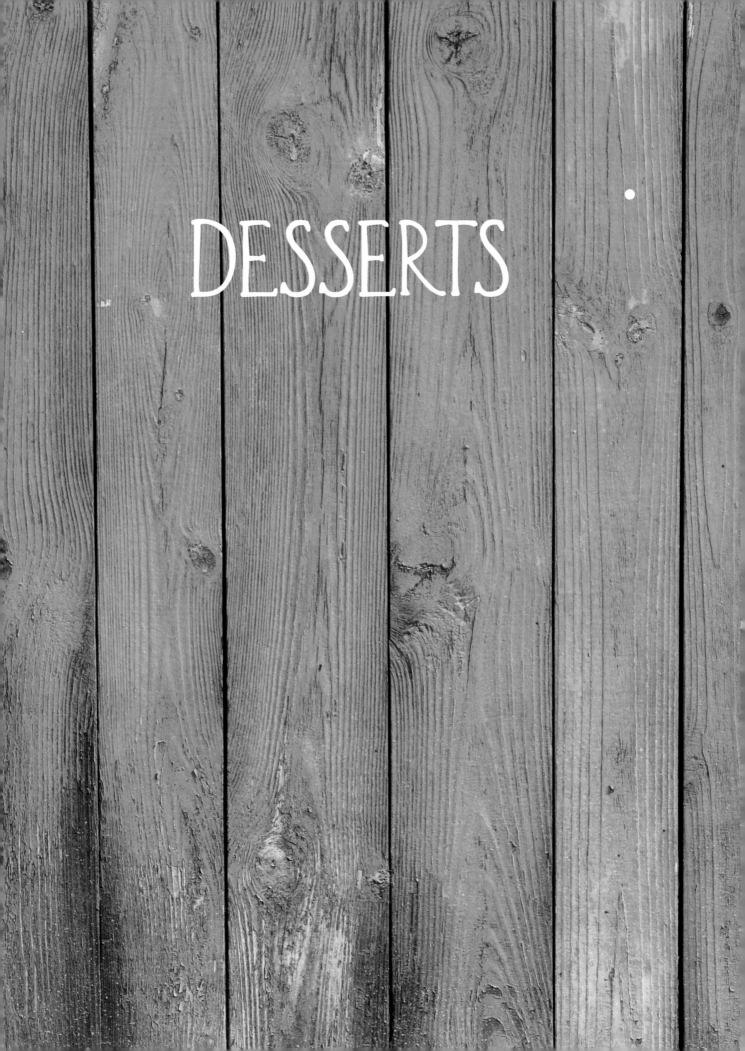

DESSERTS

BERRY SMOOTHIE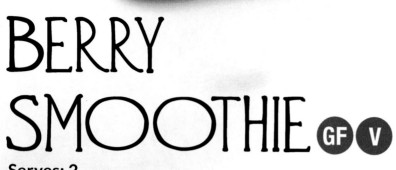

Serves: 2
Difficulty Level: 1
Cost: $$
Prep Time: 5 minutes
Cook Time: 0 minutes

SERVING SUGGESTION

TOP WITH FRESH BERRIES, IF DESIRED.

Ingredients:

1 cup frozen strawberries

1 cup full-fat unsweetened Greek yogurt (use an unsweetened coconut based yogurt for a Paleo version)

1 cup full-fat unsweetened coconut milk

1 tsp. pure vanilla extract

1 handful crushed or cubed ice

Directions:

1. Place all of the ingredients into a blender and blend until smooth.

2. Divide between two serving bowls and enjoy.

Nutrition Facts (Per Serving)

Calories: 412
Carbs: 18g
Fiber: 4g
Net Carbs: 14g
Protein: 13g
Fat: 34g

% calories from
Fat 71%
Carbs 17%
Protein 12%

MINT CHOCOLATE CHIP MILK SHAKE

Serves: 3 Difficulty Level: 1
Cost: $$
Prep Time: 5 minutes
Cook Time: 0 minutes

GF V

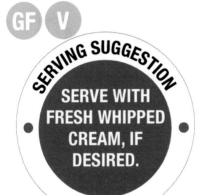

SERVING SUGGESTION
SERVE WITH FRESH WHIPPED CREAM, IF DESIRED.

Ingredients:

1 cup unsweetened almond milk

1 cup full-fat unsweetened Greek yogurt (use an unsweetened coconut based yogurt for a Paleo version)

1 avocado, pitted and peeled

1 handful fresh mint leaves

1 handful crushed or cubed ice

1 Tbsp. unsweetened chocolate chips for topping (or raw cocoa nibs) (eliminate for a Paleo version or use unsweetened raw cocoa nibs)

Directions:

1. Place all of the ingredients into a blender and blend until smooth.

2. Divide between three glasses and enjoy.

Nutrition Facts (Per Serving)
Calories: 245 Carbs: 13g Fiber: 6g Net Carbs: 7g
Protein: 9g Fat: 19g

% calories from Fat 66% Carbs 20% Protein 14%

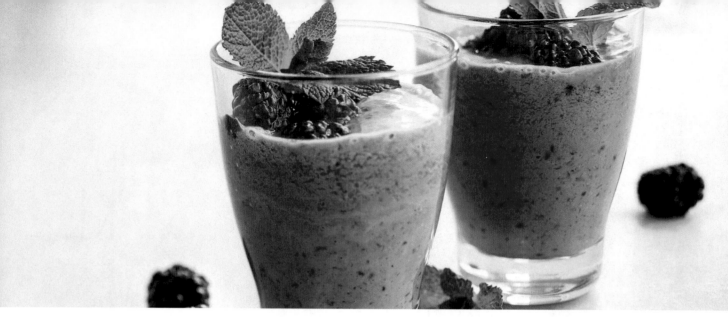

Serves: 4
Difficulty Level: 1
Cost: $$
Prep Time: 5 minutes
Cook Time: 0 minutes

Ingredients:

1 cup frozen blackberries

1 cup full-fat unsweetened Greek yogurt (use an unsweetened coconut based yogurt for a Paleo version)

1 cup full-fat unsweetened coconut milk

1 tsp. pure vanilla extract

1 handful crushed or cubed ice

1 handful fresh mint leaves (optional)

BLACKBERRY MINT SMOOTHIE (GF) (V)

Directions:

1. Place all of the ingredients into a blender and blend until smooth.

2. Divide between four glasses and enjoy.

Nutrition Facts
(Per Serving)

Calories: 214
Carbs: 10g
Fiber: 5g
Net Carbs: 9g
Protein: 7g
Fat: 17g

% calories from
Fat 69%
Carbs 18%
Protein 13%

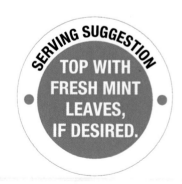

SERVING SUGGESTION
TOP WITH FRESH MINT LEAVES, IF DESIRED.

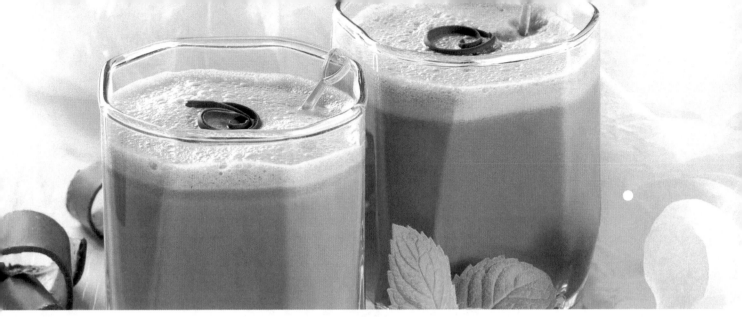

Serves: 2
Difficulty Level: 1
Cost: $$
Prep Time: 5 minutes
Cook Time: 0 minutes

COCOA LATTE SHAKE

GF **V**

Ingredients:

1 cup brewed coffee, chilled

½ cup full-fat unsweetened coconut milk

2 Tbsp. raw unsweetened cocoa powder

1 tsp. pure vanilla extract

1 tsp. ground cinnamon

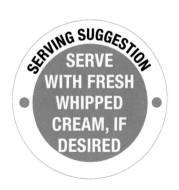

SERVING SUGGESTION
SERVE WITH FRESH WHIPPED CREAM, IF DESIRED

Directions:

1. Place all of the ingredients into a blender or food processor and blend until smooth.

2. Divide between two glasses, and top with fresh mint leaves, if desired.

Nutrition Facts
(Per Serving)

Calories: 160
Carbs: 8g
Fiber: 4g
Net Carbs: 4g
Protein: 3g
Fat: 15g

% calories from
Fat 75%
Carbs 18%
Protein 7%

VANILLA BEAN CHIA PUDDING

Serves: 4
Difficulty Level: 1
Cost: $$
Prep Time: 5 minutes + 2 hours of chilling time
Cook Time: 0 minutes

GF · **V** · **DF** · **P**

SERVING SUGGESTION

SERVE WITH FRESH MINT LEAVES, IF DESIRED.

Ingredients:

1 cup full-fat unsweetened coconut milk

¼ cup chia seeds

1 tsp. pure vanilla extract

½ cup fresh raspberries for topping

Directions:

1. Start by adding the coconut milk, chia seeds and vanilla extract to a large mixing bowl and whisk to combine.

2. Divide the mixture between four Mason-style jars and refrigerate for 2 hours or until a pudding-like consistency forms.

3. Top with fresh raspberries before serving, if desired.

Nutrition Facts (Per Serving)
Calories: 218
Carbs: 8g
Fiber: 2g
Net Carbs: 6g
Protein: 5g
Fat: 19g

% calories from
Fat 77%
Carbs 14%
Protein 9%

CHOCOLATE WALNUT FUDGE

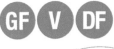

Serves: 10
Difficulty Level: 1
Cost: $$
Prep Time: 15 minutes + chilling time
Cook Time: 0 minutes

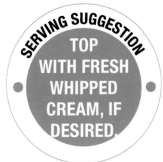

SERVING SUGGESTION
TOP WITH FRESH WHIPPED CREAM, IF DESIRED.

Ingredients:

1 cup unsweetened dark chocolate chips

¼ cup coconut oil

½ cup chopped walnuts

1 tsp. pure vanilla extract

Directions:

1. Start by adding the chocolate chips and coconut oil to a large bowl and microwave until melted.

2. Line a baking dish with parchment paper and set aside.

3. Once the chocolate mixture is melted, add the vanilla and walnuts and stir to combine.

4. Pour the chocolate mixture into the baking dish and refrigerate for 10 minutes or until set.

5. Cut into squares and enjoy.

6. Store leftovers in the refrigerator.

Nutrition Facts (Per Serving)
Calories: 199   Carbs: 14g   Fiber: 2g   Net Carbs: 12g
Protein: 3g Fat: 17g

% calories from Fat 69%   Carbs 25%   Protein 5%

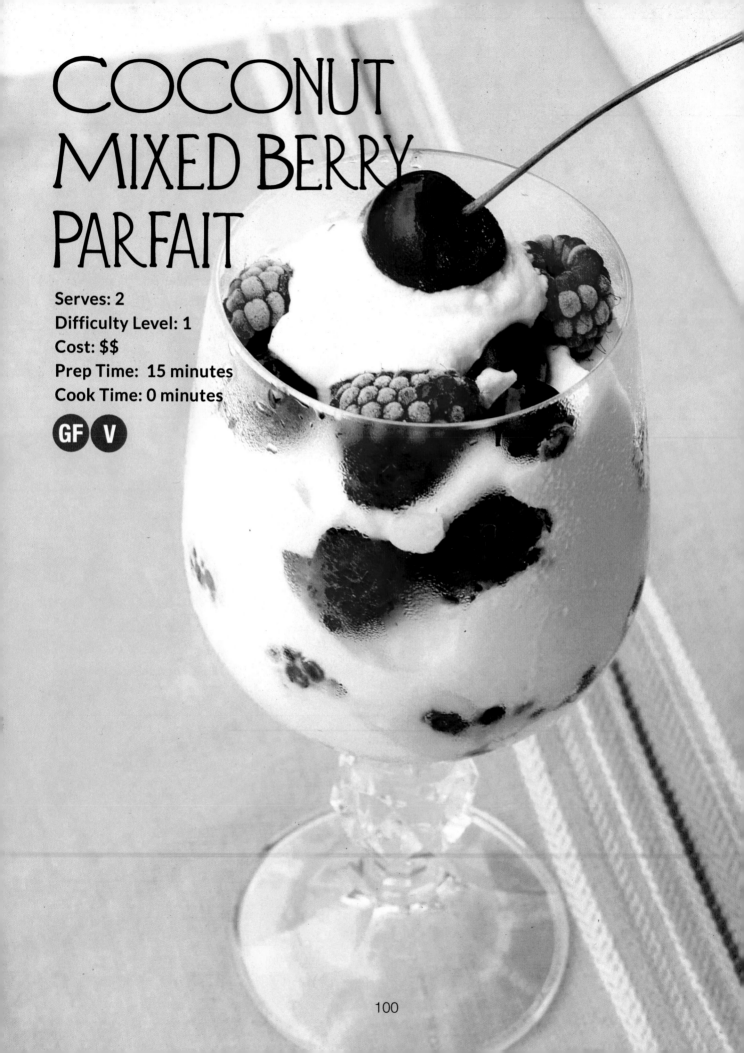

COCONUT MIXED BERRY PARFAIT

Serves: 2
Difficulty Level: 1
Cost: $$
Prep Time: 15 minutes
Cook Time: 0 minutes

GF **V**

Ingredients:

1 cup full-fat unsweetened Greek yogurt (use an unsweetened coconut based yogurt for a Paleo version)

½ cup frozen mixed berries

2 Tbsp. shredded unsweetened coconut

1 tsp. pure vanilla extract

Directions:

1. Start by adding the yogurt, shredded coconut and vanilla extract to a mixing bowl. Stir to combine.

2. Gently fold in the mixed berries.

3. Divide between two parfait glasses or serving bowls, and enjoy.

Nutrition Facts (Per Serving)

Calories: 149
Carbs: 11g
Fiber: 2g
Net Carbs: 9g
Protein: 10g
Fat: 7g

% calories from
Fat 43%
Carbs 30%
Protein 27%

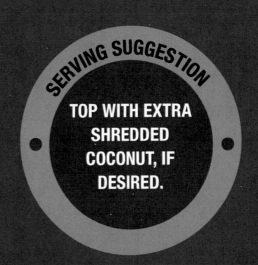

SERVING SUGGESTION

TOP WITH EXTRA SHREDDED COCONUT, IF DESIRED.

YOU MAY ALSO LIKE

Please visit the below link for other books by the author

http://ketojane.com/books

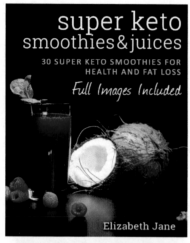

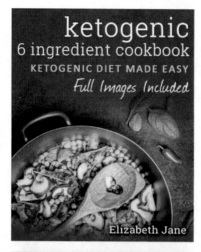

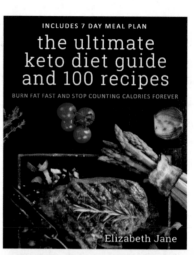

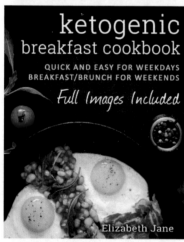

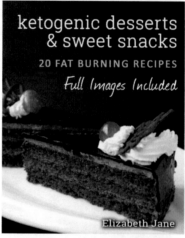

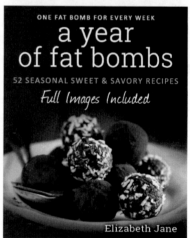

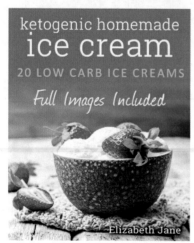

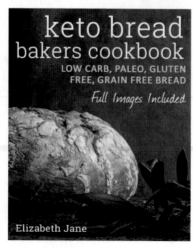

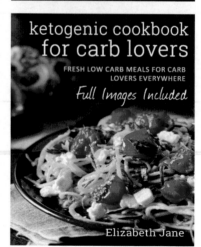

Made in the USA
Las Vegas, NV
06 April 2024